Deutsche Pharmakologische Gesellschaft

Abstracts
of the 19. Spring Meeting

March 14 – 17, 1978, Mainz

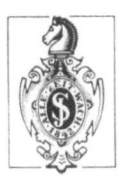

Springer International

ISBN 978-3-662-38666-8   ISBN 978-3-662-39532-5 (eBook)
DOI 10.1007/978-3-662-39532-5

Softcover reprint of the hardcover 1st edition 1978

19th Spring Meeting

Deutsche Pharmakologische Gesellschaft

Mainz, March 14 - 17, 1978

AUTHOR-INDEX

Figures = Abstract Numbers

1

INTESTINAL ABSORPTION OF COBALT AND IRON: INTERACTION AND SUBCELLULAR DISTRIBUTION
G. Becker

The absorption kinetic 10 min after administration of ^{59}Fe-$(FeCl_3)$ and ^{60}Co-$(CoCl_2)$ in increasing doses (0,5 - 1000 ng-at metal) in tied off duodenal segments of normal and iron-deficient (d) rats shows saturation characteristic for both metals. The effect of cobalt on iron absorption was studied in d rats at iron doses of 10 and 200 ng-at iron. When administring 200 ng-at iron the presence of 108 ng-at cobalt caused a reduction of iron absorption to 40 percent; excess of cobalt (1080 ng-at) diminished iron absorption to about 9 percent, whereas the uptake of iron into the mucosa did not differ from the controls. In an equal amount, however, cobalt (9 ng-at) did not diminish the absorption of iron (10 ng-at ^{59}Fe-$(FeCl_3)$. After administration of 10 ng-at ^{59}Fe-$(FeCl_3)$ together with 90 ng-at cobalt, a higher amount in the mucosa, but a diminished transfer of iron into the body was observed. The study of the time-dependence of this interaction revealed, that cobalt inhibits the release of iron from mucosal cells into the blood. This is the reason why under certain experimental conditions a storage stagnation of iron in the mucosal cells is to be seen.
The subcellular distribution of ^{59}Fe-$(FeCl_3)$ and ^{60}Co-$(CoCl_2)$ in mucosal cell homogenates of d rats after ultracentrifugation (180 000 g, 16 h, 2 - 4 ^{O}C) on a PVP/CsCl-solution shows a similar pattern for both metals. In presence of 90 ng-at cobalt the subcellular distribution of 10 ng-at ^{59}Fe-$(FeCl3)$ is not changed. This emphasizes the finding, that cobalt does not influence the uptake of iron into the mucosa.

Institut für Pharmakologie und Toxikologie der RUB, Im Lottental, D - 4630 Bochum
Institut für Pharmakologie und Toxikologie der Universität des Saarlandes, D - 6650 Homburg/Saar

2

DETERMINATION OF THE AMOUNT OF MUCOSAL TRANSFERRIN IN THE UPPER SMALL INTESTINE (DUODENUM, JEJUNUM) OF IRON DEFICIENT RATS
K. Osterloh and K. Ehrlich

Huebers et al. detected a non-ferritin protein binding iron in the mucosal cell of rats (Life Sci. 10, 1141-1148, 1971). The properties of this protein were comparable to those of plasma transferrin (ptf). Today this protein is called mucosal transferrin (mtf).
   Immunological investigations indicated a close relationship between mtf and ptf. Using antiserum against purified ptf precipitations with mtf were achieved by application of different techniques. One of these methods, the Mancini test, was found to be suitable for estimating the amount of mtf in the mucosa of iron-deficient rats. The duodenum and the upper jejunum (total: 29 cm starting with the pylorus) were used. The iron solution (^{59}Fe-$FeCl_3 \triangleq$ 200000 cpm in 2 ml 0.9% NaCl, pH 2) was filled into the tied-off segment and remained there for 10 min. Mtf was isolated by homogenisation, centrifugation (3000 g and 100000 g), column chromatography on Sepharose 6 B and ion-exchange chromatography on DEAE-Sephadex A 50.
   Using an albumin standard in all protein determinations, 8 - 11 /ug/cm mtf was found in the examined small intestine. This amount corresponds well with the yield of purified mtf found by Huebers (5.3 /ug/cm jejunum, doctors thesis Saarbrücken 1972). Chromatographical purification did not cause appreciable losses of mtf, however, mtf appeared to be lost during the concentration steps of the protein.

Institut für Pharmakologie und Toxikologie der Ruhr-Universität D4630 Bochum
Postfach 102148; Im Lottental

3

SECRETION OF THALLOUS IONS FROM THE BLOOD INTO THE GASTRO-INTESTINAL TRACT OF RATS

H.Henning and W.Forth

The secretion of thallous ions from the blood into the lumen of the stomach, the jejunum and the colon was investigated in situ on anesthetized rats (urethane, 1.25 g/kg). The method of the pendulum perfusion was used; a detailed description of the method is given. The movement of fluid was measured by aid of ^{14}C-PEG. In the stomach a net secretion of fluid was observed. The fluid volume absorbed in the jejunum and in the colon was o.o5 and o.o44 ml/cm length respectively.

After the intravenous injection of o.37 x 1o^{-8} gAt Tl/kg as ^{204}Tl-(Tl_2SO_4) the ^{204}Tl-activity in plasma fell within 2o min to about 2o% of the initial value. The halftime of this rapid phase of distribution was 8 - 9 min. A second slow phase of distribution had a halftime of 7o -75 min. Ligature of the kidneys was of no major influence on either halftime

Secretion of thallous ions into the GI-tract was measured for one hour during the slow phase of distribution of $^{204}Tl^+$-ions in the organism after the intravenous injection (dose see above). At the end of the experiment in the jejunum (5 cm length) o.35 %, in the colon (7 cm length) o.o8 % and in the stomach o.o2 % of the injected ^{204}Tl-dose was secreted. The results are discussed with respect of a possible secretion mechanism for potassium ions in the GI-tract which due to the common physicochemical properties of either ion species might be used also by thallous ions.

Institut für Pharmakologie und Toxikologie der Ruhr-Universität, D-463o Bochum, Postfach 1o2148, Im Lottental

4

CORRELATION BETWEEN THE $^{51}CrEDTA$ CLEARANCE AND THE SECRETION OF FLUID AND ELECTROLYTES UNDER THE INFLUENCE OF DEOXYCHOLATE (DC) IN THE RAT COLON.
K. J. GOERG, G. NELL, and W. SPECHT

What is the primary determinant for the changes in fluid and electrolyte movement in bile salt caused diarrhea? In tied off intestinal loops a change of motility cannot be responsible for an increase of the fluid volume. Increased mucosal cAMP content and increased adenylate cyclase activity let to the conclusion that DC is effective via an activation of the adenylate cyclase activity analogously to the action of cholera toxin. In contrast to cholera toxin, which decreases the paracellular permeability of the rat colonic mucosa, DC increases the mucosal permeability.
If this increase of epithelial permeability is responsible for the enhanced fluid production by DC, there should be a dose dependant correlation between the increase of fluid production and the increase of permeability. The rat colon was perfused in vivo. Net water, Na, Cl and K fluxes were measured and permeability was examined by determining the appearance of $^{51}CrEDTA$ in the colonic lumen after i.v. application. No change of the net water, Na and Cl fluxes and no alteration of the $^{51}CrEDTA$ clearance were found in presence of 1 mM DC. Only the K secretion was already maximally enhanced. Concentrations from 2 to 8 mM caused a dose dependent increase of water, Na and Cl secretion parallelly to an increase of the $^{51}CrEDTA$ clearance. These effects were reversibel. The correlation between the increase of fluid secretion and the increase of the epithelial permeability suggests that the effect on permeability is the predominant factor in the pathogenesis of the bile salt induced diarrhea.

Department of Pharmacology and Toxicology, University of the Saarland, D-665 Homburg/Saar.

5

INVESTIGATIONS ON THE INTESTINAL SECRETION OF DRUGS BY THE ISOLATED MUCOSA OF GUINEA-PIG COLON
U. Kilian, F. Lauterbach, and B. Pieper

The method of the isolated mucosa (F. Lauterbach, Naunyn-Schmiedeberg's Arch.Pharmacol. 297,201, 1977) was used to study cellular uptake and transepithelial permeation of labelled thiourea (Thio), digoxin (Dig), dihydro-digoxin (H2-Dig), ouabain (Ouab), N-methylscopolamine (NMScop) and ß-methylglucoside (ß-Mgl) in the colon. Mucosal pieces of 0.2 cm² had a mean wet weight (± S.E.M.) of 5.95 ± 0.13 mg (n=256). Flux chambers were filled with 0.2 ml solution and incubated at 37° for 45 min.
Contrary to the uptake of ß-Mgl, uptake of Dig,H2-Dig,Ouab and NMScop was significantly higher from the blood side. The determination of the transepithelial permeation (Table) revealed an intestinal secretion of Dig and H2-Dig which is 11-4 fold faster than observed previously in guinea-pig jejunum (F.Lauterbach in M. Kramer and F. Lauterbach: Intestinal Permeation, p. 173, Excerpta Medica, Amsterdam - Oxford 1977). In contrast to the jejunum, the difference in the transepithelial fluxes is not abolished by anaerobiosis. Furthermore, NMScop being well secreted in the small intestine (K.Turnheim and F. Lauterbach, Biochem. Pharmacol. 26, 99, 1977) crosses the colonic mucosa obviously mainly along inulin-permeable shunt pathways.This observation is regarded as evidence for the existence of several different secretory transport systems in the intestine.

Substrate	Conc.	Permeation (%)	
	µM	Lumen → Blood	Blood → Lumen
Thio	100	8.0 ± 0.20 (10)	6.1 ± 0.44 (8)
Dig	1	0.49 ± 0.04 (13)	5.6 ± 0.33 (14)
H2-Dig	1	0.48 ± 0.05 (8)	7.7 ± 0.63 (10)
Ouab	1	0.25 ± 0.08 (8)	0.57 ± 0.16 (8)
NMScop	10	0.84 ± 0.30 (5)	0.69 ± 0.15 (5)
ß-Mgl	1000	0.53 ± 0.06 (11)	0.71 ± 0.11 (9)

Institut für Pharmakologie und Toxikologie der Ruhr-Universität, Im Lottental, D-4630 Bochum

6

BINDING OF DRUGS TO MUSCLE TISSUE: DRUG INTER-ACTIONS   B. Fichtl, H. Kurz, I. Wachter, A. Ziegler

Skeletal muscle of rabbits was homogenized with equal volume of isotonic phosphate buffer pH 7.0. The binding of drugs (10^{-4} M/l) was determined by ultrafiltration. The concentration of the unbound drug (c_u) increased significantly ($p < 0.01$) in the presence of a second drug in equimolar concentrations in the following cases:

Drug	Influenced by	% Change of c_u
Phenprocoumon	Tolbutamide	+ 23
Phenprocoumon	Phenylbutazone	+ 10
Quinine	Promethazine	+ 22
Morphine	Phenylbutazone	+ 11
Chlorpromazine	Suramin	+ 85
Quinine	Desipramine (10^{-3} M/l)	+ 27
Nitrosalicylic acid	Phenylbutazone (10^{-3} M/l)	+ 14

On the other hand the concentration of the unbound amount of sulfadimethoxine decreased in the presence of phenylbutazone by 15%.
Insignificantly or not influenced was the binding of nitrosalicylic acid (by atropine, chlorpromazine), sulfadimethoxine (by quinine, sulfinpyrazone), phenprocoumon (by chlorpromazine), nitrofurantoin (by phenylbutazone), thiopental (by phenylbutazone), mecamylamine (by thiopental, nitrofurantoin), tolbutamide (by phenylbutazone), quinine (by chlordiazepoxide, phenylbutazone), morphine (by promethazine), chlorpromazine (by thiopental).

Pharmakologisches Institut der Universität München, Nussbaumstrasse 26, D-8000 München 2

7

PROBENECID EFFECTS ON DISTRIBUTION AND ELIMINATION OF BENZYLPENICILLIN IN THE RAT
H.Bergholz, R.R.Erttmann, and K.H.Damm*

Previous studies of the effects of probenecid on penicillin distribution indicate that inhibition of renal secretion is not the only effect by which elevated plasma levels can be explained (Ziv and Sulman, Arch.int.Pharmacodyn. 207, 373, 1974). We have investigated the effect of 50 mg /kg b.w. probenecid on distribution and bile excretion of C_{14} benzylpenicillin (bp) 5-90 min after i.p.application of 25 mg/kg b.w. Radioactivity was measured by scintillation counting and bp concentration was calculated by use of internal standards. It was found that under probenecid the concentration of bp in plasma, cerebrospinal fluid and skeletal muscle increased up to 2- to 3fold over the controls. At the same time the values in liver and kidney were lowered from 30 to 70 percent of the controls and consequently the tissue/plasma ratio of bp was decreased from 6.2 to 2.8 in the liver and from 6.3 to 2.3 in the kidney. The bile excretion of bp was not significantly influenced by probenecid. But the half time of bp calculated was increased from 24.9 min to 33.2 min by probenecid while the volume of distribution and the total clearance were lowered considerably (from 312 to 128 ml and from 7.4 to 2.85 ml/min, respectively). The results indicate that besides the inhibition of renal tubular secretion other effects do contribute to the elevated plasma levels of bp following probenecid application.

Pharmakologisches Institut der Universität
D-2000 Hamburg 20, Martinistraße 52
*Universitätskinderklinik FU D-1000 Berlin 19

8

RESORPTION RATE OF Mg AND Al FROM ANTACIDA REMEDIES - INFLUENCES ON THE DISTRIBUTION OF ELECTROLYTES AND TRACE ELEMENTS
H. P. Bertram

The polyvalent cations in antacids cannot be regarded as non-absorbable. In chronic renal failure Al-containing drugs are used to control hyperphosphataemia. Resorbed Al is discussed to play a role in dialysis encephalopathy syndrome. We examined patients (n = 68) with renal insufficiency and daily intake of 5 g $Al(OH)_3$. The plasma-Al of the treated patients was significantly higher (3,06 umol/l) than in the control group (o,87). In the same specimens Zn shows a slight decrease, Cu an elevation.

The amount of Al-absorption by means of flameless atomic absorption spectrophotometry was also measured after a single therapeutical dose in normal individuals. To 15 healthy volunteers different antacids were given: $Al(OH)_3$; mixture of $CaCO_3$+$Al(OH)_3$+$Mg(OH)_2$; complex basic Al-Mg-carbonate. Evaluation of the kinetic values was made for each person separately under standard-conditions with special regard to food. Nearly all probands showed a distinct Al-Absorption. Since the urinary Al-levels are not directly correlated with the plasma-Al, beside the single Al-estimation in urine at different times a 24-h-urine collection was made to reveal the total renal Al-output. Maximum of resorption was reached after 2 - 3 hrs. Mg-containing antacids caused a distinct increase in Mg-plasma-levels, but still remaining in the normal range. Possible interactions with electrolytes and trace elements lead to the determination of Ca, Na, K, Fe, Cu, Zn, Cr in the same specimens. In order to get more detailed information on possible pathogenetic processes it seems to be useful to look for a "metal fingerprint" in biological samples.

Institute of Pharmacology and Toxicology, University of Münster, Westring 12, D-4400 Münster

9

DISPOSITION AND ANTICOAGULANT ACTIVITY OF THE ENANTIOMERS OF PHENPROCOUMON IN PHENOBARBITAL PRETREATED RATS
W. Schmidt

The purpose of this study was to assess in rats the effect of enzyme induction on the stereoselective disposition and anticoagulant activity of phenprocoumon.

The experiments were performed in untreated and phenobarbital pretreated (75 mg/kg for 4 days) male inbred Wistar-Lewis rats following single i.v. injections (0.6 mg/kg) of S(-) or R(+)phenprocoumon.

Phenobarbital pretreatment caused an increase in the elimination rate and a decrease in the total anticoagulant effect per dose of both enantiomers. The plasma concentration-effect relationship of the enantiomers was not significantly affected by pretreatment with phenobarbital. The synthesis rate of prothrombin complex activity prior to the injection of phenprocoumon was higher in phenobarbital pretreated rats than in control rats, indicating that phenobarbital induces the synthesis of clotting factors.

The intrinsic elimination rate constant and to a less degree also the fraction of dose in the liver of both enantiomers increased after pretreatment with phenobarbital. The former was the result of enzyme induction, the latter due to the increase in liver weight. There was no difference between S(-) and R(+)phenprocoumon in the relative changes of the pharmacokinetic parameters after pretreatment with phenobarbital.

Pharmakologisches Institut der Universität Mainz, Obere Zahlbacher Str. 67, D-6500 Mainz

10

IN VIVO STUDIES ON THE INTERACTION BETWEEN PHENPROCOUMON AND ACETYLSALICYLIC ACID OR PHENYLBUTAZONE   H.-M. Brinkmann, H.H. Jess, K.-U. Seiler

After intravenous injection of a loading dose of ^{3}H-phenprocoumon (P) to rabbits, the drug was infused for a period of 10 hours. By this procedure a steady state concentration for total P (C_{SST}) of 19 ug/ml plasma and for free P (C_{SSF}) of 3.4% of C_{SST} was attained immediately after injection. Interstitial fluid (IF) was drawn from tissue cages implanted subcutaneously according to D. CHISHOLM et al. (Brit.med.J. 1, 569-573, 1973). After 7 to 10 hrs the total concentrations of P in this fluid amounted to 55% of the corresponding plasma value, the C_{SSF} being 4.3% of the C_{SST} in the IF. 5 hours after starting the application of P acetylsalicylic acid (AS) or phenylbutazone (PB) were also administered by combination of a loading dose and subsequent infusion. The C_{SST} of AS and of PB were in the range of 100 ug/ml and 70 ug/ml plasma, respectively. Immediately upon addition of AS or PB the free fraction of P in the plasma increased to 4.3% and 5.5% resp., and in the IF to 6,4% (AS) and 6.1% (PB), and were permanently maintained. In spite of the fact that both AS and PB reduce the protein binding of P in plasma and IF, opposite effects were observed with respect to C_{SST} and C_{SSF}. Upon addition of AS the C_{SST} and C_{SSF} in both compartments were reduced to lower levels (75%). This may be explained by diffusion of displaced P into the intracellular space, where the protein binding appears not to be influenced by AS. After addition of PB, however, the C_{SST} was found to be unaltered in plasma and IF, while the C_{SSF} were considerably increased. It may be assumed that the PB will intracellularly compete with protein bound P thus increasing the concentration of free P also within the cells. Therefore a concentration gradient for free P does not exist between extra- and intracellular space. Hence, after administration of PB the free P concentrations are elevated in all compartments accessible for P and PB.
Department of Pharmacology, University of Kiel, D 23 Kiel, Hospitalstrasse 4 - 6

11

EXCRETION OF AN ANALOGON OF CLONIDINE COMPARED WITH CLONIDINE IN RATS. U. Gundert-Remy and E. Weber

An analogon of clonidine substituted in the benzene ring with bromide instead of chloride was given to female rats in a dose which has no effect on the blood pressure. The substance was randomly tritiated (specific activity 3.76 mCi/mg; NEN). The radioactive purity amounted to 96 -97 %.
In animals with cannulated bile duct 22.5 ± 2.1% of the radioactivity were excreted with the bile. Over 9o % of the total radioactivity was found to run with an Rf-value of o.o7 in the systeme used. The Rf-value of the parent compound was 0.85 using thin layer chromatography. After giving clonidine the biliary excretion of the radioactivity amounted to 15.2 ± 2.1% of the dose. About 8o% were not the parent compound. The bile cannulated rats excreted 37.6 ± 10.0 % of the dose of the clonidine analogon with the urine. Only a small part of the radioactivity was due to the parent substance. The figure for clonidine was 48.1 ± 9.9% of the given radioactivity in the urine from which about 8o% was the parent compound.
In rats with ligated bile duct 66.2 ± 5.2% were excreted urinary when the clonidine analogon was given. The main part of the radioactivity accounted for metabolites. The urinary excretion of clonidine was 74.o ± 7.1% under the same conditions. 7o% were unchanged. The clonidine analogon was handled in the same manner as clonidine with respect to the biliary excretion. Comparing the urinary excretion a greater part of the radioactivity was found as unchanged substance after clonidine.
Abt.f. Klin.Pharm. Med. Univ.Klinik, 69 HD

12

A UNIVERSAL AND SENSITIVE METHOD FOR GAS CHROMATOGRAPHIC DETERMINATION OF VOLATILE SUBSTRATES AND METABOLITES
W. Dünges, and K. Kiesel

The concentration of solutes from aqueous solutions in the µl range is still a problem in gas chromatographic trace analysis (e.g. J.S. Fritz, Acc. Chem. Res. 10, 67, 1977).
Standardized extraction and extract concentration procedures are described for the g c analysis of volatile substances in sub-ml amounts of aqueuous solutions. Extraction by stirring (P.L. Kirk, Adv. Chrom. 5, 79, 1968) was combined with concentration under partial reflux (K. Beyermann et al., Z. Anal. Chem. 251, 289, 1970). Technical improvements have resulted in clean blanks and high reproducibility (W. Dünges and K. Kiesel in "Assay of biological samples for drugs and other trace compounds" E. Reid, ed., in press).
O-nitrotoluene, o-nitro-anisole, phenol and benzylalcohol in ppM amounts were extracted from 250 µl water with ethyl acetate. The volume of the extracts was reduced to 5 µl. Glass capillary g c according to K. Grob was then performed. The g c peak ratios: compounds/internal standards were similar to those from test runs. The recovery rates were 60 to 80%. Six complete pre-chromatographic experiments were performed in 80 min.
Presented are: the possibilities of the method and detailed working instructions.
The g c determination of the above and related compounds in nanogram amounts seems of general methodological interest, e.g. in pharmacological studies of microsomal hydroxylation.

Pharmakologisches Institut der Universität Mainz, Obere Zahlbacher Str. 67, D-6500 Mainz

13

DRUG BINDING PROPERTIES OF TYROSINE-MODIFIED HUMAN SERUM ALBUMIN   K.J. Fehske, and U. Wollert

Human serum albumin (HSA) has only a small number of specific binding sites for drugs. There are facts indicating that tyrosine residues may be involved in these binding sites. Thus we modified HSA with tetranitromethan, a reagent specific for tyrosine residues in proteins. As derived from an UV-absorption quotient three albumins with a degree of modification of two, five and eight residues per molecule were obtained. Only for the albumin with eight residues modified a small reduction of ordered secondary structure was found.

The drug binding properties of the modified albumins were investigated by circular dichroism measurements and by equilibrium dialysis. The induced Cotton effects of most of the drugs investigated were reduced e.g. diazepam, tetrazepam, chlordiazepoxid, iophenoxic acid, 8-anilino-1-naphthalene sulfonic acid and sulfadimethoxine. The extrinsic Cotton effects of phenylbutazone and flufenamic acid bound to tyrosine-modified HSA are increased compared to unmodified HSA. The circular dichroism spectra of warfarin, dicumarol and some biliary contrast agents show fundamental changes when bound to HSA or tyrosine-modified HSA.

It was found by equilibrium dialysis that the affinity of diazepam and L-tryptophan to the benzodiazepin binding site of HSA is strongly reduced after modification of tyrosine residues while the number of binding sites remains unaffected. It is suggested that tyrosine residues are located in or very close to the stereospecific benzodiazepine binding site. The location of this binding site in the primary structure of HSA is discussed.

Pharmakologisches Institut der Universität Mainz, Obere Zahlbacher Str. 67, D-6500 Mainz

14

THE INTERACTION OF INTRAVENOUS AND ORAL BILIARY CONTRAST AGENTS WITH SERUM ALBUMINS   W.E. Müller

The binding of two homologous series of oral and intravenous biliary contrast agents to human and bovine serum albumin was investigated using the gel filtration technique and circular dichroism measurements.
All intravenous compounds are bound to human serum albumin via one high affinity and several low affinity binding sites. Within the concentration range investigated, about three to five high affinity binding sites for the oral compounds were found on the human serum albumin molecule. In general, the intravenous compounds have a greater affinity for human serum albumin than the oral compounds. No significant differences were found for the binding of the oral compounds to human or bovine serum albumin, while the intravenous compounds have a higher affinity for bovine than for human serum albumin.
The binding of most of the intravenous and oral biliary contrast agents to human and bovine serum albumin generates extrinsic Cotton effects. The positions of the maxima and the intensities of the induced Cotton effects vary for the compounds and the two albumins. The observed differences give some evidence for small differences of the complex formations of the compounds with human and bovine serum albumin. The extrinsic Cotton effects are depending on the pH of the solution. The reason seems to be the conformational change of the albumins between pH 8-9 rather than changes of the complex formation.
The significance of the different serum albumin binding of the oral and intravenous biliary contrast agents for the pharmacokinetics of the drugs and their uptake into the liver is discussed.

Pharmakologisches Institut der Universität Mainz, Obere Zahlbacher Str. 67, D-6500 Mainz

15

BIOCHEMICAL PROPERTIES OF PLASMA MEMBRANES FROM CANDIDA TROPICALIS GROWN ON GLUCOSE OR HEXADECANE
G.F.Fuhrmann, H.Schneider and A.Fiechter

Candida tropicalis cells are able to assimilate hydrocarbons as single carbon source. In continuous culture experiments following a substrate change from glucose to hexadecane, an adaption phase occurred (H.Hug, H.W.Blanch and A.Fiechter, Biotechnol.Bioeng. XVI, 965, 1974). Therefore, possible structure changes of the plasma membrane before and after the adaption period were examined.
Plasma membrane vesicles were isolated from mechanically disrupted cells by filtration, differential centrifugation and aggregation of mitochondria. For chemical analysis of the membranes the plasmatic content of the vesicles was released by cytolysis. The purity of the plasma membranes was more than 95% as judged by electron microscopic criteria and biochemical examinations of marker enzymes.
After the adaption phase from glucose to hexadecane the following changes in the plasma membrane structure have been measured: a change of the plasma membrane protein pattern as revealed by SDS polyacrylamide gel electrophoresis, an increase of the cytochrome b5 content, induction of aldehyde- and alcoholdehydrogenase, changes in the fatty acid composition and a shift of the isoelectric point to higher pH values by cell electrophoresis technique. The mechanism of hexadecane transfer will be discussed.

Department of Pharmacology and Toxicology, School of Medicine, Lahnberge, D-3550 Marburg, Germany and Institute of Microbiology, Swiss Federal Institute of Technology, Zürich, Switzerland.

This work was supported by S.N.S.F. grant No.: 3.622/0.75

16

ALTERATIONS OF LYSOSOMES BY AMPHIPHILIC DRUGS

U. Gidion and O. Wassermann

During our studies on drug-induced impairment of phospholipid metabolism the influence of several amphiphilic drugs on lysosomes has been studied, and the alterations detected have been analysed isolating these organelles.
Rats (SD, male, 250 g) were treated with chloroquine, mepacrine (400 mg/kg, p.o.) or chlorphentermine (2 x 50 mg/kg, i.p.) for 3 days. Already after this short treatment lipid and drug deposits are visible in the liver lysosomes using fluorescence/polarisation microscopy according to Staiger (Experientia 30, 385, 1974).

By means of differential and sucrose density gradient centrifugation liver lysosomes were concentrated in certain fractions and characterized by electron microscopy and by determination of three lysosomal enzymes. The drug-modified lysosomes have accumulated the drugs and showed both a distinctly lower density and alterations in the lipid pattern compared to controls.

Supported by Deutsche Forschungsgemeinschaft (Wa 284/9)

Department of Toxicology, University of Kiel, D-2300 Kiel Hospitalstrasse 4-6, Germany

17

INFLUENCE OF NICLOSAMIDE AND PHENPROCOUMONE ON THE LEVEL OF ENERGY PHOSPHATES AND SELECTED SUBSTRATES OF GLYCOLYSIS IN RAT LIVER
A.Schütz, G.Malorny, R.Huljus, U.Wendisch

In preliminary investigations we determined the intravenous LD_{50} of both decoupling substances (niclosamide 8.25 mg/kg, phenprocoumone 55 mg/kg). We established a distinct increasing during 10 min to 1 h. We gained the liver sample by the double hasket (two sledges) and stop freeze method of Faupel et al.(Arch.Biochem.Biophys. 148, 509,1972). We cooled the samples between aluminium blocks extremly cooled by liquid nitrogen (-195° C). We determined the anoxia time of the liver. This time is necessary to calculate the level of our substrates back to the zero point. In the following alkaline and acid decomposition we pretreated the samples for the photometric tests. We measured following substrates in 3 hours: ATP, ADP, AMP, glucose 6 phosphate, lactate, pyruvate, citrate, and glycogen. The substrates of the adenylate system changed in a typical kind after the administration of decoupling substances. ATP was decreased in the first 30 min. ADP and AMP increased in the same time. During the tests we established an enhancement of glycolysis. The glycogen level changed in correspondence to glucose 6 phosphate. The citrate level increased by niclosamide administration distinctly.

Pharmakologisches Institut der Universität Hamburg, Martinistraße 52, D-2000 Hamburg 20

18

MODE OF ACTION OF TERBUFIBROL (INN), A NEW HYPOLIPEMIC AGENT R. Löser, I. Steffen and M. Kussmaul

To investigate the mode of action of the new hypolipoproteinemic compound Terbufibrol (4'-[3-(4'-t-butylphenoxy)-2-hydroxy-propoxy]benzoic acid) the effect on hepatic HMG-CoA reductase (EC 1.1.1.34) and 7-α-hydroxylase (EC 1.14) activity was studied in comparison to Clofibrate (CPIB). Male Wistar rats were conditioned to controlled day-time feeding and then pretreated orally with the test drugs. In these animals Terbufibrol was at least twice as active as CPIB lowering serum total cholesterol (TC). HMG-CoA reductase was assayed in 10 000xg and 7-α-hydroxylase in 18 000 xg supernatants of liver homogenate by following the incorporation of 14C-acetate (14C-mevalonate) into cholesterol (Ch) and the conversion of 14C-Ch to 7-α-hydroxy-Ch, respectively.

In contrast to CPIB, Terbufibrol effected a dose-dependent, max. 6-fold stimulation of HMG-CoA reductase, without interfering with the diurnal rhythm of this enzyme activity. The effect was the same after 4,14,and 25 days of treatment. Dexamethasone completely blocked this stimulation of HMG-CoA reductase, while having no effect on the TC-lowering action of Terbufibrol. Therefore the stimulation of this enzyme must be secondary to the lipid lowering activity of this drug. Terbufibrol and CPIB both inhibited 7-α-hydroxylase, i.e., an increase of the catabolic rate of Ch cannot account for the TC-reducing action. On the other hand, repeated doses of Terbufibrol increased basal bile flow and the hepatic bile acid pool size.

It is concluded that Terbufibrol acts either by inhibiting a key step of lipoprotein (LP) synthesis or interfering with the release of LPs into the circulation. The increase of bile acid pool size is considered to be independent of the hypolipemic action but it may be one of the secondary factors affecting the above enzyme activities.

Biochemische Pharmakologie, Klinge Pharma GMBH & Co., D 8 München 40

19

PHARMACOLOGY OF TERBUFIBROL (INN), A NEW HYPOLIPEMIC AGENT
R. Zschocke, G. Hofrichter, H. Grill, H. Hampel, H. Liehn

The pharmacology of Terbufibrol (4'-[3-(4'-t-butylphenoxy)-2-hydroxy-propoxy]benzoic acid) was studied in comparison to Clofibrate(CPIB).Both drugs had very similar acute toxicities in rats and baboons. Hypolipemic/hypolipoproteinemic properties were evaluated in a test system described previously (Zschocke et al.,In:Prot.Biol.Fluids,25,Pergamon, 1978,p.535) employing normal ♂ rats and ♂ baboons as well as several experimental hyperlipoproteinemias in both species. In rats Terbufibrol was 2-5 and in baboons 10 times more effective than CPIB reducing serum total cholesterol (TC). The triglyceride lowering activity was twice that of CPIB. In baboons Terbufibrol had no effect on VLDL turnover, which was increased by CPIB (Intralipid test). Prep.ultracentrifugal analysis showed that Terbufibrol had a significantly greater effect on VLDL-TC in rats and LDL-TC in baboons than CPIB, resulting in a max.increase of the ratio HDL-TC/VLDL-TC by +113% (CPIB: +54%) and the ratio HDL-TC/LDL-TC by +132% (CPIB: -33%), respectively. In long-term treatment max.hypolipemic response was maintained over 4 weeks in rats and 8 weeks in baboons; equi-effective doses of Terbufibrol produced less hepatomegaly than CPIB. Increases in liver lipids were similar with both drugs except for TC, which was increased respectively decreased during Terbufibrol and CPIB treatment. Repeated doses of Terbufibrol increased basal bile flow and hepatic bile acid pool size in rats. Neither drug affected the lithogenic index in baboons. In further studies Terbufibrol showed moderate antilipolytic activity in vivo (ca.1/2 Nicot.Acid) and inhibition of ADP-and collagen-induced platelet aggregation in vitro (ca.ASA); it had no estrogenic activity and did not increase cholesterol precursors in plasma of rats and baboons. Concluding, Terbufibrol appears to be a promising new drug for the treatment of hyperlipoproteinemias.

Pharmakologische Forschung, Klinge Pharma GMBH & Co., D 8 München 40

20

PREMATURE INDUCTION OF THE DECIDUAL REACTION AFTER CYCLOPHOSPHAMIDE TREATMENT IN THE RAT H. Spielmann & R. Herken

After treatment of pregnant rats or mice during the preimplantation period with cyclophosphamide (CPA), the embryos are retarded and die during organogenesis. Previous studies using both in vivo and in vitro approaches have shown that the embryos are affected by CPA-treatment of the mother already before implantation (J. Embryol. exp. Morph. 41, 65, 1977; Nature 270, 54, 1977). The same investigations indicated an inhibition of the decidual reaction of the uterus during organogenesis after CPA-treatment before implantation. - To elucidate to what extent effects of the early CPA-treatment on the decidualization of the uterus are involved in the delayed embryolethal effect, the course of the decidual reaction was investigated during the implantation period after CPA-application. On day 3 of gestation rats were treated with a single s.c. injection of 60 mg/kg CPA. Between days 4 and 7 the uteri were examined light microscopically. In addition, the labelling index of the stroma cells on day 4 (preimplantation)and day 6 (postimplantation) was determined after a ^{3}H-thymidine pulse, On day 4 the increase in the labelling index of the uterine stroma cells 24 h after CPA-application on day 3 (40% as compared to 7% in controls) as well as the light microscopical findings of an increased cell number and a reduction in the size of the intercellular spaces underneath the uterine epithelium suggest a premature decidual reaction. On day 6 of gestation the percentage of stroma cells which had differentiated into decidual cells was increased after CPA-treatment when compared to untreated controls. It is, therefore, concluded that the transformation of stroma cells into decidual cells is induced prematurely by CPA-application before implantation. Furthermore, the percentage of necrotic stroma cells increased between days 4 and 7 in CPA-treated animals, eventually leading to a reduction in the amount of decidual tissue.
This work was supported by DFG grants (Sfb 29). Institut für Toxikologie und Embryonal-Pharmakologie, Freie Universität Berlin, Garystr. 9, D-1000 Berlin 33, West-Germany.

21

EFFECT OF STEROID SEX HORMONES ON THE DEVELOPMENT OF EARLY MOUSE EMBRYOS *IN VITRO*   H.-G. Eibs and U. Jacob-Müller

In vitro culture methods of early mammalian embryos allow an evaluation of pharmacological effects after early maternal treatment on embryonic development (Nature 270, 54, 1977). After maternal administration of the gestagens cyproterone acetate (CA) or medroxygesterone acetate (5-50 mg/kg s.c.) on day 2 of pregnancy (p.c.) we obtained mouse morulae and blastocysts on day 3 p.c. and cultured them *in vitro* for 120 h. The number of embryos per mother and the blastocyst/morula quotient was not affected. During the *in vitro* culture the rate of embryos that hatched, attached to the surface of the petri dish, and developed a differentiated trophoblast layer remained constant. However, differentiation of the inner cell mass (ICM) into 2 germ layers was inhibited irrespective of the dose (76% in controls; 44% after treatment). The additional application of estrogen on day 2 p.c. (0.03 µg estron/mouse) did not alter the rate of embryos developing 2 ICM germ layers but reduced the number of blastocysts on day 3. However, the application of a single dose of 0.03 µg estrogen/mother only inhibited the embryonic development in culture. Blastocyst culture in the presence of estrogen either without or after maternal gestagen treatment inhibited hatching and attachment of the blastocysts and all subsequent developmental steps. After treatment of mice with CA (5-100 mg/kg) on day 1 and 2 p.c. teratological investigations were performed at term (day 17). As a preliminary result the rate of exencephalic fetuses was significantly increased from 0.4% (spontaneous rate) to 2.1% after treatment. This effect was not dose-dependent. This result might be interpreted as a co-teratogenic effect whose mechanism remains to be explained. To test this hypothesis, mice were treated with CA on day 2 p.c. and subsequently on days 9,10,11, or 12 with the teratogens cyclophosphamide and methylnitrosourea. So far only a significant reduction in the fetal weight at term could additionally be induced by CA.

Supported by DFG grants, Inst. f. Toxikologie & Embryonal-Pharmakologie, Freie Universität, Garystr. 9, 1 Berlin 33.

22

PHARMACOKINETICS OF PHENAZONE IN THE RAT - THE CLASSICAL PHENAZONE DETERMINATION REVISITED   Schüppel,R.; J.Böttcher; H. Bäßmann

Besides Phenazone, some of its metabolites are also subject to nitrosation, owing to a free C-4-position. It has further been demonstrated, that 3-HO-phenazone, 3-carboxy-phenazone and nor-phenazone are present, at least in part, in the free form in blood, urine and liver perfusate of the rat. Therefore, specificity of the classical phenazone determination (BRODIE et al. JBC 179, 25-1949) may be questioned.

Starting from authentic material, spectra of 4-(iso-)-nitroso-derivatives of the above metabolite were compared with that of the parent compound. As expected, all of them showed a peak at 350 nm, the molar extinction coefficient being very similar. Correspondingly, extracts of biological material from rats being dosed with phenazone (liver perfusate, blood, urine) after nitrosation can be shown by TLC-scanning to contain 4-nitroso-derivatives of either phenazone and the metabolites mentioned. Similar patterns were found using 14-C-labeled phenazone, synthezised in our laboratory. It proved impossible to remove these contaminants by refined extraction procedures.

Therefore, a method was elaborated for the specific determination of phenazone using quantitative TLC and densitometric scanning (ZEISS KM-3). Comparing elimination kinetics of phenazone in the rat with both TLC-scanning and the nitrosation reaction, there were marked differences between half-life time and related data, e.g. T/2 (TLC-scan): 1.0 hr vs. T/2 (nitrosation): 2.5 hrs Nitrosation reaction, therefore, seems inadequate as an analytical tool in pharmacokinetic studies using phenazone as a model drug in the rat.

Dpt.Pharmacol.TU Braunschweig,D-33-Braunschweig

23

BINDING SITES WITH DIFFERENT AFFINITY TO PENICILLINS IN STAPHYLOCOCCAL MEMBRANES
H.Keppeler and W.Bruns

In cytoplasmic membranes of Escherichia coli and Bacillus subtilis there are multiple penicillin binding components. In contrast, only one type of them was assumed to be in staphylococci, although there is some evidence for the existence of two different binding sites in this species (BLUMBERG, P.M., STROMINGER, J.L., Bact. Rev. 38, 291, 1974). Therefore we studied the binding of a number of penicillins to the cytoplasmic membrane of Staph.aureus H by measuring the uptake of ^{14}C-benzylpenicillin after preincubation with the nonradioactive penicillins.

Two types of binding sites with different affinity were found for the isoxazolyl-penicillins as well as for methicillin and ampicillin. On the other hand the binding components for benzyl-penicillin, carbenicillin, azlocillin and mezlocillin are homogeneous. In the following the binding constants of oxacillin are compared to those of benzylpenicillin.

	n	K
Oxacillin	11.3 (n_1)	7.0×10^{-8} (K_1)
	7.8 (n_2)	9.0×10^{-5} (K_2)
Benzyl-penicillin	20.8	2.0×10^{-8}

n: number of binding sites (nmoles/g protein
K: dissociation constants (moles/l)

The differences in binding may be caused by two separate proteins or by a single protein being located in various sections of the membrane.

Department of Pharmacology, University of Köln, Gleuelerstrasse 24, D 5000 Köln 41

24

INVESTIGATIONS ON THE MEMBRANE ACTIVITY OF CYTO-STATIC METHYL HYDRAZONES R.Braun, W.Dittmar, W.-D. Gassel[+]

N'-Methyl-N'-ß-chloroethylhydrazones show cytostatic, immune suppressive and immune stimulative activities according to their dosage and way of application. These hydrazones cause a strong inhibition of the uptake of nucleosides into Ehrlich-ascites-carcinoma cells (EAC), but no interference with DNA or RNA polymerizing systems could be observed. Therefore, an attack on the cell membrane was supposed.

Experiments for studying structure-activity-relationships show that an aziridinium ion, which is formed immediately from the hydrazones in the cell membrane, is responsible for the observed effects but not an alkylating reaction. Thus, analogous hydrazones, in which the ß-chloroethyl group was replaced by other groups leading to a partial positive charge at the N'-moiety without the ability of alkylation, also show cytostatic effects in vivo and inhibited uptake of nucleosides in vitro. Furthermore, no reactions with SH-groups and guanosine could be detected at physiological conditions. The number of SH-groups, at the surface of EAC determined by the DTNB-method, increased to 180 % of the control under the influence of ß-chloroethyl hydrazones. Probably, this finding is caused by a rearrangement after incorporation of the hydrazones into the cell membrane.

However, if dimethyl sulfoxide (DMSO, 0,5% v/v) is present in the medium, the tumor cells die rapidly as compared with the control under the influence of the ß-chloroethyl hydrazones. Similar effects could be observed on stem cells of bone marrow of mice (C 57 BL), when they were incubated in the presence of a clone stimulating factor (CSF) in dependence of the concentration of CSF, a strong decrease could be observed in the presence of DMSO.

Institute für Pharmakologie und Toxikologie und [+]Medizinische Poliklinik, Universität Marburg, Lahnberge, D-3550 Marburg/Lahn

25

VIRAZOLE (RIBAVIRIN) A CYTOSTATIC AGENT. J. Arendes,
R. K. Zahn and W. E. G. Müller

Virazole (1-ß-D-ribofuranosyl-1,2,4-triazole-3carboxamide,riba-
virin) is a synthetic triazol nucleoside with a broad spectrum of
antiviral activity. But virazole affects the metabolism not only of
virus infected cells. Virazole strongly inhibits the cell proliferation of mouse lymphoma cells (L 5178y), which were not infected
with DNA- or RNA-viruses. Starting with 3×10^3 cells/ml and an
incubation period of 72 hr, the drug reduces the cell proliferation
to 50 % (= ED_{50} concentration) in a concentration of $4,7 \mu M$.
Virazole acts cytostatically up to 3 times the ED_{50} concentration.
The cytostatic effect of virazole can be abolished by guanosine,
xanthosine and inosine but not by adenosine. These data indicate
that virazole interferes with the guanosine metabolism.
Incorporation studies with radio-labeled precursors into DNA,
RNA and protein in intact L 5178y cells showed, that the incorporation rates are inhibited by virazole. Already 2 hr after incubation with the drug the amount of polyribosomes decreases. In the
presence of virazole, the pool sizes of GTP and dGTP are drasti-
cally reduced.
Chemically synthesized virazole 5'-triphosphate was tested in
different DNA- and RNA polymerizing systems. No effects were
found on eukaryotic DNA polymerase α and ß, eukaryotic RNA
polymerase I and II, and eukaryotic poly (A) polymerase. Therefore
the inhibition of nucleic acid syntheses must be attributed to the
depletion of GTP and dGTP in the virazole-treated cells.

Institut für Physiologische Chemie, Universität Mainz, Duisberg-
weg, D-6500 Mainz

26

DIHYDRODIOL DEHYDROGENASE: AN IMPORTANT ENZYME
IN DIHYDRODIOL-EPOXIDE PATHWAY - MEDIATED
BENZO(A)PYRENE MUTAGENICITY.
Bentley, P., Vogel, K., Glatt, H. R., Platt, K. and
Oesch, F.

Benzo(a)pyrene is metabolized to two major groups of mutagenically reactive metabolites: Monofunctional epoxides and dihydrodiol-epoxides. Various monooxygenase forms catalyze the
various pathways at very different rates. In metabolic situations where the contribution by dihydrodiol-epoxides is small,
epoxide hydratase represents a very efficient protective system.
However, in situations where the mutagenic effect is predomi-
nantely due to dihydrodiol-epoxide, the effect of epoxide
hydratase is complicated and weak. We have now obtained
evidence that a dihydrodiol dehydrogenase represents an efficient protective system in the latter situation. The enyzme
was purified to homogeneity and the pure enyzme added to
systems generating mutagenically active benzo(a)pyrene metabolites by the presence of various monooxygenase forms. In
situations where epoxide hydratase had only weak effects, dihydrodiol dehydrogenase afforded efficient protection and vice-
versa.

Acknowledgment: This work was supported by DFG.

Institute of Pharmacology, University of Mainz, Obere
Zahlbacher Straße 67, D-6500 Mainz

27

ON THE ROLE OF UNSPECIFIC CARBOXYLESTERASES
(EC 3.1.1.1) IN THE METABOLISM OF ACETYLSALICYLIC
ACID AND PROCAINE W. Block, S. Kaßpohl and C. Keck

Unspecific carboxylesterases (CE) are involved in drug metabolism
by hydrolyzing ester and amide bonds. Their significance in vivo,
however, compared to the contributions of other esterases is unknown so far in most cases. Since previous studies (Block and
Wassermann, 1976 and 1977) provided evidence of the high specificity of bis-p-nitrophenylphosphate (BNPP) as an irreversible inhibitor of CE in the rat, the influence of BNPP-pretreatment on the
fate of (carboxyl-^{14}C)procaine (P) and of acetyl(carboxyl-^{14}C)
salicylic acid (ASA) was investigated. 12 hrs after i.p. inj. of 100
mg BNPP/kg b.w. (or of 0.9% NaCl=controls) 10 mg of ^{14}C-P
or ^{14}C-ASA were i.p. applied to rats (Wistar, female, 150 g).
During 24 hrs 20.1% (12.3%) of the dose were found in the urine
as unchanged P and 2.8% (0.7%) as unchanged ASA (values in
brackets=controls). In mice the toxicity of P is augmented by
BNPP-pretreatment, the LD_{50} decreased by a factor of 1.8. After
preincubation of mouse liver homogenate with 10^{-4}M BNPP (30 min,
37°C) the "procaine esterase" was almost totally inhibited. Using
a continuous spectrophotometric test, 40% of the procaine hydrolyzing activity of mouse plasma and 60% of the ASA hydrolyzing
activity of rat serum were found sensitive to BNPP. Values for
v_{max} and k_M of controls and of the non-BNPP-sensitive fractions
are provided by Lineweaver-Burk plots. In human plasma or serum
neither procaine esterase nor ASA esterase was inhibited after
preincubation with BNPP; this is in good agreement with the known
fact, that human plasma contains no CE, and provides an additional argument for the high specificity of BNPP. - The application
of BNPP in toxicologic and teratologic studies on the molecular
mechanisms of the known side-effects of ASA appears promising.
Supported by the DFG.

Department of Toxicology, University of Kiel, D-2300 Kiel,
Hospitalstrasse 4-6, Germany

28

PHARMACOLOGICAL CHARACTERIZATION OF BAY G 5421,
A GLUCOSIDASE INHIBITOR FOR THE TREATMENT OF
CARBOHYDRATE-DEPENDENT METABOLIC DISORDERS.

W. Puls, U. Keup, H.P. Krause, and G. Thomas

BAY g 5421[*] delays starch as well as sucrose
digestion in the small intestine by inhibiting
glucosidases involved in the hydrolysis of oli-
gosaccharides. As a consequence in loading tests
with both carbohydrates the blood glucose and
serum insulin increments are reduced in animals
and in man. The ED 50 is approximately 0.5-3 mg
BAY g 5421/kg per os.
In feeding experiments with genetically obese
and hyperlipaemic rats the inhibitor reduced
body weight gain to the level of non-obese rats
and diminished the serum triglyceride and cholesterol concentration. The carcass lipid-content was markedly reduced and the carcass pro-
tein-content was increased. Fenfluramine reduced the body weight gain without affecting the
carcass lipid-content. Administration of clofibrate lowered the serum cholesterol. Nicoti-
nic acid and phenformin had no significant effect on the above mentioned parameters.

Conclusions: BAY g 5421 seems to be a suitable
compound for the improvement of carbohydrate
tolerance in diabetics and for reduction of serum and adipose tissue lipids in hyperlipaemic
and obese people.
*)
0-[4,6-Dideoxy-4-[[1S-(1,4,6/5)-4,5,6-trihydroxy-
3-hydroxymethyl-2-cyclohexene-1-yl]-amino]-α-D-
glucopyranosyl]-(1 $\longrightarrow$ 4)-0-α-D-glucopyranosyl-
(1 $\longrightarrow$ 4)-D-glucopyranose

Institute of Pharmacology, Bayer AG, Box 101709,
5600 Wuppertal 1

29

ON THE MECHANISM OF DIGITOXOSIDE CLEAVAGE OF DIGITOXIN IN RAT LIVER

A.Schmoldt, C.Rohloff, and H.F.Benthe

Previous studies have shown that digitoxin (Dt-3) is metabolized by rat liver microsomes to digoxin (Dg-3) and bis- and mono-digitoxosides of born digitoxigenin (Dt-2 and Dt-1) and digoxigenin (Dg-2 and Dg-1). Moreover, more lipophilic glycoside(s) were found in vitro and in vivo (in bile after iv.injection). Presumably, these are formed by oxidation of the sugar chain (Schmoldt et al.,Biochem.Pharmacol.$\underline{24}$,1639,1975). No metabolism could be measured in vitro in the absence of NADPH or O_2 suggesting that unchanged digitoxosides cannot be hydrolyzed by microsomal enzymes.

The aim of the present study was to investigate the structure of the more lipophilic metabolites and their possible part for digitoxin metabolism. Synthesized 3'''(")(')-dehydrodigitoxosides of digitoxigenin (Dt-3ox,Dt-2ox,and Dt-1ox,resp.)correspond exactly to lipophilic metabolites of Dt-3,Dt-2,and Dt-1. The terminal 3-dehydrodigitoxose can be split off by liver microsomes under anaerobic conditions. 110 pmoles Dt-3ox and Dt-2ox were cleaved by 1 mg microsomal protein/min. However,for Dt-1ox only a rate of 15 pmoles/min was measured (substrate conc.50 µM).

From these results it can be concluded that:
1. digitoxosides can be cleaved only after oxidation of the terminal sugar. 2. The free genin cannot be found in vivo because of the higher stability of Dt-1ox. Therefore Dt-1 is the main substrate for conjugating enzymes.

Pharmakologisches Institut der Universität Hamburg, Martinistraße 52, D-2000 Hamburg 20

30

TYPE I- SUBSTRATE BINDING AND OXIDASE FUNCTION OF MICROSOMAL CYTOCHROME P-450.

G. HEINEMEYER and A.G. HILDEBRANDT

The stoichiometry of hydroxylation reactions represents the sum of hydroxylase and oxidase activity (Biochem.Soc.Trans.$\underline{3}$,807(1975),Arch.Biochem.Biophys.$\underline{180}$, 343(1977)). The latter can be expressed by formation rates of H_2O_2. As the amount of H_2O_2 produced varies among others by the addition of substrates, it was postulated (B.B.R.C. $\underline{54}$,968(1973)) that oxidase, oxygenase and peroxidase function associated with cytochrome P-450 are controlled by the spin state of cytochrome P-450, which can be expressed by e.g. the spectral change elicited by type I binding substrates such as hexobarbital.

H_2O_2 production and spectral binding to hepatic microsomal cytochrome P-450 increase in parallel upon addition of similar amounts of hexobarbital:

	K_m (H_2O_2)	K_s (hexobarbital)	n
rabbit	0.32 + 0.25	0.12 + 0.05	5
guinea pig	0.46 + 0.32	0.35 + 0.1	5

Accordingly, the magnitude of hexobarbital binding and rates of H_2O_2 formation correlate significantly in each species tested.

Furthermore, spectral binding (E_{max}) and rates of H_2O_2 (V_{max}) correlate with concentrations of cytochrome P-450. While spectral binding is independent on species, rates of H_2O_2 formation correlate to cytochrome P-450 content but change within species tested, probably due to limitations in electron transport or membrane differences.

It is suggested that modification of cytochrome P-450 by hexobarbital leads to a spectral change (type I) which correlates with oxidase activity rather than formation of an ES complex during hydroxylation reactions.

Dept. of Clin.Pharmacol. Free University, Klinikum Steglitz, 1 Berlin 45, Hindenburgdamm 30

31

SPECTRAL INTERACTIONS WITH CYTOCHROME P-450 PRODUCED BY XENOBIOTICS IN ISOLATED ADULT RAT HEPATOCYTES

B.C. Sweatman*, K.J. Netter* and J.W. Bridges

Type I and II binding spectra have been demonstrated in isolated adult rat hepatocytes suspended in 2.5% gelatin. The type I spectral binding constants for hexobarbital and naphthalene were similar to those observed in rat hepatic microsomes. On addition of safrole to the hepatocytes an initial type I binding spectrum was observed which developed with time into a spectrum with 427 nm (major) and 460 nm (minor) peaks, which is characteristic of the formation of a safrole metabolite-cytochrome P-450 complex. These findings show a) that cytochrome P-450 exists in cells at least in part, in the oxidised state b) that cytochrome P-450 in situ is not fully bound to endogenous materials, and c) that putative toxic metabolites shown previously with microsomal preparations are likely to be formed readily in vivo.

*Institute of Pharmacology and Toxicology, University of Marburg, Lahnberge, D-3550 Marburg/Lahn

Dept. of Biochemistry, University of Surrey, Guildford, U. K.

32

STUDIES ON THE CYTOCHROME P-450-PRODUCT COMPLEXES FORMED DURING THE METABOLISM OF NN-DIMETHYLANILINE

P. Hlavica and G. Aichinger

The oxidative metabolism of NN-dimethylaniline (DMA) by partially solubilized cytochrome P-450 from rabbit liver is associated with the appearence of a double Soret difference spectrum with absorbance bands at 424 and 448 nm. These spectral changes closely resemble those observed during the metabolism of a series of methylenedioxyphenyl compounds and amphetamines by liver microsomal fractions (M.R. Franklin, Xenobiotica $\underline{1}$, 581, 1971; M.R. Franklin, Drug Metab. Dispos. $\underline{2}$, 321, 1974). Addition of the primary reaction products from DMA, i.e. N-methylaniline and NN-dimethylaniline N-oxide, to haemoprotein preparations fortified with NADPH results in the formation of a 424 and 440-447 nm chromophore, respectively, suggesting a potential relationship between these spectral changes and the C- and N-oxidation of DMA. This view is supported by the ability of a series of factors such as modification of pH, metabolic alteration by n-octylamine, induction by phenobarbital or 3-methylcholanthrene, removal of lipid from the enzyme preparations and preincubation of purified cytochrome P-450 at 37°C in the absence of NADPH to influence the formation of the metabolite complexes and the enzymic C- and N-oxidation of DMA to comparable extents.

Pharmakologisches Institut der Universität München, Nussbaumstr. 26, D-8000, München 2, Federal Republic of Germany

33

EFFECT OF ANTIOXIDANTS ON MICROSOMAL ENZYMES OF RAT LIVER
R. Kahl

Rat diet was supplemented with butylated hydroxytoluene (BHT), butylated hydroxyanisole (BHA) or ethoxyquin (EQ) for 14 days, and hepatic microsomal epoxide hydratase (EH) and monooxygenase were subsequently studied in vitro. The antioxidants increased EH activity. The increase was marked with BHT (factor 3) and EQ (factor 4) and was paralleled by an increase in a protein band on SDS polyacrylamide gels which migrated together with purified rat hepatic EH. A slight but nonsignificant increase in cytochrome P450 content and a moderate increase in ethoxycoumarin deethylation and cytochrome b_5 content was also observed while aryl hydrocarbon hydroxylase (AHH) activity was not elevated. Irreversible binding of metabolically activated benzo(a)pyrene (BP) to calf thymus DNA was slightly reduced when catalyzed by antioxidant-stimulated microsomes. The cytochrome P450 population was similar to that found in phenobarbital (PB)-stimulated liver as jugded from preferential inhibition by and high affinity binding of metyrapone. The antioxidants also inhibited AHH activity in vitro in PB-stimulated microsomes, but not in 3-methylcholanthrene (MC)-stimulated microsomes.
Mixed induction with dietary antioxidants and intraperitoneally administered MC led to similar induction of EH as in the absence of MC. However, AHH activity and covalent binding of BP were decreased under these conditions. This shift in the microsomal enzyme pattern may be related to the protective effect of antioxidants against chemical carcinogenesis (Wattenberg, L.W., J.Natl.Cancer Inst. 48, 1425, 1972).

Department of Pharmacology, Section of Toxicology, University of Mainz, Obere Zahlbacher Str. 67, D-6500 Mainz

34

SUBSTRATE SPECIFICITY OF RABBIT LIVER MONOOXYGENASE INDUCED BY PCBs.   Th. Wolff

Exposure of rats to PCBs induces the two groups of hepatic monooxygenases that are inducible by phenobarbital (PB) or methylcholanthrene (MC)(Alvares et al., PNAS 70,1321,1973). By contrast, in rabbit liver a number of monooxygenase activities which are enhanced by PB neither respond to the application of PCBs nor to MC (Wolff et al.,Biochem.Pharmac. 26,783,1977). This suggests that in rabbit liver the PCB-inducible monooxygenase might be of the cytochrome P-448 form. To verify this assumption, 3 reactions were studied which are stimulated by MC treatment. Rabbits were treated with a single oral dose of 50 mg/kg PCB (CLOPHEN A 50) on 5 consecutive days. Liver microsomes were isolated 3 days thereafter. PCB treatment enhanced N-hydroxylation of acetylaminofluorene (AAF) 8-fold, and acetanilide and zoxazolamine hydroxylation almost 3-fold. A 4-fold increase of AAF and a 2-fold increase of acetanilide and zoxazolamine metabolism was observed after MC treatment (2x20 mg/kg) indicating a close relationship between PCB and MC mediated induction.
The P-448 dependent metabolism of the three substrates in PCB or MC induced rabbit liver microsomes suggests a particular affinity of the enzyme to a common structure of these compounds. Due to resonance stabilisation of the N-acetylgroup with the aromatic ring the molecular conformation of AAF and acetanilide resembles a benzoxazole ring which is a constituent part of zoxazolamine. Possibly, this benzoxazole like structure is responsible for the substrate specificity of hepatic cytochrome P-448 in rabbits.

Gesellschaft f. Strahlen- u. Umweltforschung, Abtlg. Toxikologie, D-8042 Neuherberg/München.

35

STRAUB-PHENOMENON DURATION AS A MEASURE OF ACTIVITY OF DRUG-METABOLIZING LIVER ENZYMES
F. E. BEYHL

The duration time of the STRAUB phenomenon in mice after morphine administration is dose-dependent; it is linear to the logarithm of the dose of morphine.
Administration of α-hydroxy-α-ethylbutyryl diethylamide (HOE 17 879), a known inhibitor of hepatic microsomal drug-metabolizing mixed-function oxidases, in a dose of 150 mg/kg i. p., 30 minutes prior to a standard dose of 6 mg/kg morphine. HCl i. v., prolongs STRAUB phenomenon duration time up to 190.1 % of the control value, whereas aminopyrine N-demethylase, papaverine O-demethylase and guaiacol glycerol ether ring hydroxylase activities in liver are decreased to 30.9, 19.6, and 56.8 %, resp., of the control values.
Pretreatment of mice with phenobarbital for four days in a daily dose of 75 mg/kg, leads to a decrease of the STRAUB phenomenon duration time after a standard dose of 6 mg/kg of morphine hydrochloride to 78.3 % of the control value and to increases of the enzyme activities of aminopyrine N-demethylase, morphine N-demethylase, and papaverine O-demethylase to 610.0, 150.8, and 228.0 % resp. of the control values.
Therefore the authors propose the use of STRAUB phenomenon duration time determinations as an in vivo assay method for the assessment of the liver's capability to metabolize foreign compounds, similar as hexobarbital sleeping time measurements but with restriction only to mice.

HOECHST A.G., D - 6230 Frankfurt (M) 80

36

THE POSSIBLE ROLE OF THE ENZYME PEROXIDASE FOR THE ORGANOTROPIC TOXICITY OF DIETHYLSTILBESTROL
M. Metzler and J.A. McLachlan

In-utero exposure to the synthetic estrogen diethylstilbestrol (DES) has been associated with teratogenic lesions in the lower genital tract of women and with vaginal carcinoma later in life. The Müllerian duct is considered the target tissue for the organotropic toxicity of DES, but the reasons for its susceptibility are at present not well understood.
From our studies on the metabolism of DES we propose to consider the metabolic activation of DES through a peroxidase-mediated oxidation as a possible mechanism of organotropism. This hypothesis is based on the facts that
(1) oxidation of DES by peroxidase in-vitro leads to β-dienestrol, which is also a major DES metabolite in-vivo.
(2) the intermediates of the peroxidase-mediated formation of β-dienestrol are the semiquinone and quinone of DES, which are chemically reactive compounds. In fact, nonextractable binding of 14C-radioactivity to albumin and deoxyribonucleic acid was found after in-vitro incubation of these macromolecules with 14C-DES and peroxidase from horse radish.
(3) peroxidase activity according to the literature occurs preferentially in tissues depending on estrogens for growth, and is inducible by estrogens.
It is thus conceivable that DES induces peroxidase in the cells of the Müllerian duct and is oxidized by this enzyme to reactive intermediates capable of damaging cellular macromolecules.

Institute of Toxicology, University of Würzburg, D-8700 Würzburg, Versbacher Landstraße 9

37

INFLUENCE OF Mn^{2+}-IONS ON ADRENALINE OXIDATION AND LIPID PEROXIDATION CATALYSED BY RAT LIVER MICROSOMES OR BY ISOLATED NADPH-CYTOCHROME C REDUCTASE, H. Kappus[+] and J.B. Schenkman

It is well established that adrenaline is oxidised by rat liver microsomes to adrenochrome. Furthermore, complexes of Mn^{2+}-ions with adrenaline can readily be autoxidised. We incubated rat liver microsomes (2 mg protein/ml), adrenaline (0.2 mM) and $MnCl_2$ in presence and absence of NADPH. Adrenochrome was formed depending on the $MnCl_2$-concentration in both cases. The Mn^{2+}-induced adrenochrome formation rate in absence of NADPH increased from 1 mM to 50 mM $MnCl_2$ (40 nmol adrenochrome/ml/min). In presence of NADPH, however, the adrenochrome formation rate which amounted normally to about 22 nmol/ml/min increased between 1 μM and 0.1 mM $MnCl_2$. At saturation conditions with $MnCl_2$ (0.1 mM) 118 nmol adrenochrome/ml/min were formed. The complex of Fe^{2+}-ions with adrenaline was oxidizable by NADPH-dependent enzymes, whereas it was stable against autoxidation. If $MnCl_2$ was used at 0.1 mM Fe^{2+}-ions inhibited the NADPH-dependent Mn^{2+}-induced adrenochrome formation to 50 % at 0.1 mM $FeCl_2$. In contrast to the Mn^{2+}-induced autoxidation of adrenaline, the NADPH-dependent Mn^{2+}-induced adrenochrome formation was inhibited by 10 U/ml superoxide dismutase (SOD). Microsomal NADPH-dependent lipid peroxidation induced by Fe^{2+}-ions was inhibited to 50 % by 0.1 mM $MnCl_2$, but not by SOD (10 U/ml). All effects of $MnCl_2$ on adrenaline oxidation and lipid peroxidation in the microsomal system could also be observed during incubations with isolated NADPH-cytochrome c reductase.

Department of Pharmacology, Yale University Medical School, New Haven, Ct., 06510, U.S.A.
[+]Present address: Institut für Toxikologie der Universität, Wilhelmstraße 56, D 7400 Tübingen

38

EVIDENCE FOR TWO DISTINCT TERTIARY AMINE OXIDASES
J.W. Gorrod, L.A. Damani, and L. Patterson

Communication withdrawn

Department of Pharmacy, Chelsea College (University of London) Annexe, 271 King Street, London, W6 9LZ, U.K.

39

THE METABOLISM OF SULPIRIDE IN THE RAT K. Dross

Biotransformation and distribution of sulpiride (SP) was studied using carbonyl-14-C labelled (SP A) as well as 3,4-pyrrolidin-14-C labelled substance (SP B). Purification and isolation of labelled metabolites was performed by preparative TLC. A spectrophotometric TLC scanning procedure was applied to compare isolated compounds to chemically prepared putative metabolites. After 5o mg SP A/kg (2o μCi/rat) ip. 5o% of injected radioactivity was found in urine, 3o% in feces. 74% of urinary and 55% of fecal radioactivity is due to unchanged SP, i.e. about 33% of given SP is metabolised. O-demethylated SP represented 9% of total excreted radioactivity, while the N-desethylated compound amounted to 2%, the 5-oxo-pyrrolidin-SP to 4%, the O-demethyl-5-oxo-pyrrolidin-SP to less than 1%. Another 1o% were coupled to a compound not identified but most likely demethylated. Almost identical autoradiographs were got from bidimensional separations of urine from rats which received either SP A or SP B, i.e. only minute amounts of SP were metabolised by hydrolysis of the amide-linkage. Relative 14-C-concentrations one hour after ip.-application (2o mg SP/kg) of liver/serum/brain were 1oo/1o/1, contents of other tissues(kidney, lung, spleen, muscle, intestine) ranged between 3o and 5o. The percentual fraction of unchanged SP/total radioactivity was lowest in liver and intestine (36 resp. 44%), medium in kidney, lung, serum and spleen (56%, 6o%, 63%, 72%) and highest in brain (93%). It seems unlikely that a metabolite contributes to the central action of SP.

C. und O. Vogt - Institut für Hirnforschung der Universität Düsseldorf, Moorenstr. 5, D-4ooo Düsseldorf.

40

METABOLIC DEGRADATION OF CLONIDINE   S. Darda, H.-J. Förster, and H. Stähle

^{14}C-clonidine was administered orally to dogs (Beagles) for 5 days. 6 radioactive substances eliminated with the urine could be isolated. They were identified by mass spectrometry and comparison with synthetic material. The presence of unchanged clonidine, p-hydroxy-clonidine, and dichlorophenylguanidine was confirmed and 3 new metabolites were detected: 1-(2,6-dichloro-4-hydroxyphenyl)guanidine; 2-[(2,6-dichlorophenyl)imino]imidazolidine-4-one, and 2-[(2,6-dichloro-4-hydroxyphenyl)-imino]imidazolidine-4-one. The cleavage of the imidazolidine ring and the hydroxylation of the phenyl ring are the two principal routes of metabolism. In an additional experiment, the metabolic patterns in the urine of man, rat, and dog were compared after a single oral dose of labelled clonidine. It could be demonstrated that the 6 identified compounds were eliminated by all 3 species, the relative amounts, however, were different. Man eliminated clonidine mainly in the unchanged form. In the urine of the rat a considerable amount of the parent drug could be detected but the metabolites predominated. Of the 3 species investigated the dog metabolized clonidine most readily with dichloro-phenylguanidine as its main metabolite.

Biochemical, Analytical, and Chemical Departments, C.H. Boehringer Sohn, D-6507 Ingelheim

41

REDUCTIVE METABOLISM OF P-NITROBENZOIC ACID AND NITRAZEPAM IN THE ISOLATED PERFUSED RAT LIVER IN THE PRESENCE OF ETHANOL   H.G. Jonen

Reductive metabolism of aromatic nitro compounds has been shown to play a minor role under aerobic conditions and to reach maximal activities under anoxia (Jonen-Kern et al., Xenobiotica, in press). We have shown that in the presence of ethanol maximal activities can be obtained even under aerobic conditions.
Nitro reduction was studied in isolated perfused rat livers with a recirculating hemoglobin free medium. Using nitrazepam as the substrate (1mM) there is considerable aerobic formation of 7-acetylamino derivative, but only small amounts of unconjugated 7-amino derivative are formed (cf. Bartošek et al., Europ. J. Pharmacol. 11, 378, 1970). Under anoxia as well as aerobically in the presence of ethanol (38mM) a 6-8-fold increase in the formation of free 7-amino derivative in the perfusate is seen whereas the formation of the 7-acetylamino derivative remains almost unchanged. When p-nitrobenzoic acid was the substrate (2mM) anoxia as well as addition of ethanol led to a 7-fold enhancement of free p-aminobenzoic acid and to a 2-3-fold increase of conjugated p-aminobenzoic acid. The concentrations of free and conjugated reduced metabolites in the liver exhibited only slight increases under anaerobic conditions as well as in the presence of ethanol, irrespective of the substrate.
Perfusion experiments with carbon monoxide in which only the anaerobic reduction but not the aerobic ethanol mediated reduction of p-nitrobenzoic acid was inhibited, point to the involvement of different cellular compartments (endoplasmatic resp. cytoplasmatic) in the two processes. The amount of aerobic reduction of p-nitrobenzoic acid in the presence of acetaldehyde (35mM) which even supersedes the effect of ethanol possibly indicates the requirement of ethanol oxidation in the enhancement effect.

Department of Pharmacology, University of Mainz,
Obere Zahlbacher Straße 67, D-6500 Mainz

42

NUCLEOTIDE KINETICS IN PHASE II OF DRUG BIOTRANS-FORMATION AS MEASURED BY ^{31}-P-NMR-SPECTROSCOPY
A. Stier, S. Finch, and T. Slater

^{31}P-Fourier-NMR-spectroscopy using a Bruker-WH 270-spectrometer was applied as a direct, qualitative and quantitative analytical technique to the measurement of the kinetics of uridine diphosphate glucuronic acid (UDPGA), uridine diphosphate (UDP), uridine monophosphate (UMP) and of phosphate (P) associated with the glucuronidation of drugs. During glucuronidation of p-nitrophenol (PNP) in incubations of microsomes from phenobarbital stimulated rabbits a stoichiometry of the overall reaction

$$UDPGA + PNP \rightarrow UMP + P + PNPGA \quad (1)$$

was observed.
The reaction

$$UDP \rightarrow UMP + P \quad (2)$$

was faster than reaction (1).
EDTA (10^{-3} M) totally inhibited reaction (2). The same substance influenced reaction (1) quantitatively, but not qualitatively, particularly no intermediate formation of UDP could be detected.
In the presence of the detergent Triton X 100 and EDTA the reaction

$$UDPGA + PNP \rightarrow UDP + PNPGA \quad (3)$$

was observed.
The results are discussed in relation to
a) tranversal orientation of the glucuronyl transfer within the microsomal membrane and
b) functional linkage of microsomal enzyme reactions.

Max-Planck-Institut für Biophysikalische Chemie
D-3400 Göttingen

*Dept. of Biochem., Brunel University, Uxbridge, UK

43

THE EFFECT OF CONJUGATION ON UPTAKE AND SECRETION OF LIPOPHILIC COMPOUNDS BY ISOLATED HEPATOCYTES   M. Schwenk

Isolated rat hepatocytes were used to investigate important factors that influence the transhepatic transport of lipophilic compounds (ethinyl estradiol, estrone and naphthol). Cellular uptake, intracellular metabolism and secretion of the metabolites were determined simultaneously.
Methods: Cells (1mg prot./ml) were incubated with radiolabelled compounds for 20 min. At various times cells were separated from the extracellular medium. Both cellular space and extracellular medium were analysed for the concentrations of the original compounds and their metabolites.
Results: All 3 lipophilic compounds were rapidly taken up (40 - 70 %) by hepatocytes. The compounds were metabolized in cells to water soluble conjugates, which were secreted in saturable active processes.
Ethinyl estradiol (1 µM) is metabolized to ortho-hydroxylated products. Water soluble metabolites were released, mainly in the form of glucuronides. Estrone (1 µM) is converted to glucuronides (about 60 %) and sulfates (about 30 %). Intracellular conjugation of naphthol is very rapid. The conjugates are trapped in the cells, indicating that conjugation is much faster than active secretion. The effect of substrate concentration and of various inhibitors on these kinetics is demonstrated. The value of this model for the investigation of hepatic transport is discussed .

Institute of Toxicology, University of Tübingen,
Wilhelmstr. 56, D-7400 Tübingen

44

HEPATIC UPTAKE, METABOLISM AND SECRETION OF ESTRONE SULPHATE   V. Lopez del Pino

Estrone sulphate (ES) is a major transport form of estrogens. The pharmacokinetics of ES are described in this presentation. (^{3}H) ES (10 mg dissolved in 0,9 % NaCl) was injected intravenously into the rat. It disappeared rapidly from the blood, with a half life of less than 5 minutes. The biliary secretion of ES reached a maximum at 15 minutes. This peak was accompanied by a choleretic effect. In 60 minutes about 20 % of the injected radioactivity was recovered in the bile. Biliary radioactivity appeared mainly as a glucuronide conjugate (about 60 %) and to a lesser extent as sulphate conjugates. In the isolated perfused liver 80 % of the radioactivity was eliminated in the bile in 60 minutes. The pattern of the whole conjugates was similar to that found in the whole animal.
Hepatic transport was further characterized by the use of isolated hepatocytes. ES uptake exhibits saturability, inhibition by antimycin A, mersalyl and taurolithocholate. Uptake is Na - dependent, and is inhibited by ouabain. These features are consistent with carrier-mediated transport. In the cell the sulphate ester is rapidly cleaved and metabolized at the steroid moiety. The intracellular metabolites are preferentially conjugated to glucuronides. These conjugates are secreted in an energy-dependent step.

Institute of Toxicology , University of Tübingen,
Wilhelmstr. 56, D-7400 Tübingen

45

STUDIES WITH ISOLATED LIVER CELLS: KINETICS AND METABOLISM OF BROMOSULFOPHTHALEIN (BSP)
L.R. Schwarz

Uptake, conjugation with glutathione and secretion of bromosulfophthalein (BSP) was studied in isolated liver cells.

Hepatocytes (3 mg protein / ml) were preincubated for 10 min in Leibovitz L-15 medium before 35-S-BSP was added to the suspension. To stop the reaction and to separate the cells from the medium, hepatocytes (0.5 mg protein) were centrifuged into silicon oil and immediately frozen. Conjugated and nonconjugated BSP was separated and determined by TLC and liquid scintillation counting.

When cells are incubated with 25 nMol 35-S-BSP/ ml nearly all BSP is taken up from the supernatant within 20 min. Simultaneously, conjugated BSP appears in the medium at a rate of about 0.12 nMol/min x mg protein. Throughout the first 25 min half the intracellular BSP is conjugated, thereafter the percentage of the BSP metabolite increases. Free as well as conjugated BSP reach their intracellular maximum after about 10-15 min. - The metabolic inhibitor, Antimycin A, diminishes the rate of formation and secretion of conjugated BSP. Conjugation of BSP is also affected by styrolepoxide and tetrachloride which are known to lower the glutathione level.
These data indicate that isolated hepatocytes are a useful model to study drug kinetics.

Dept. of Toxicology, Gesellschaft für Strahlen- und Umweltforschung, D-8042 Neuherberg.

46

SENSITIVE RADIO-ASSAYS FOR THE DETERMINATION OF MICROSOMAL UDP-GLUCURONYLTRANSFERASE IN HUMAN LIVER BIOPSY SPECIMENS K.W. Bock, E. Huber, and D. Josting

UDP-glucuronyltransferase (GT) can accurately and conveniently be determined in 0.2 - 1 mg of liver biopsies using ^{14}C-1-naphthol as substrate. After incubation (37°C, pH 7.4, 0.5 mM 1-naphthol, 3 mM UDP-glucuronic acid, 5 mM $MgCl_2$) > 98% of free 1-naphthol is removed from the incubation mixture by one extraction with $CHCl_3$ and the radioactivity of the glucuronide is determined in the aqueous phase. Two K_M-values were found for 1-naphthol. This may suggest that the substrate is glucuronidated by more than one GT. In biopsies from patients with no histological liver damage and no exposure to enzyme inducers native and Brij 58-activated GT was 0.11 $\pm$ 0.04 (n=7) and 0.87 $\pm$ 0.23 (n=18) μmol/ min/g liver, respectively. GT in biopsies from patients with cholelithiasis and histological pericholangitis was significantly decreased whereas GT from patients with alcoholic liver damage was unchanged or slightly increased. GT (^{14}C-morphine as substrate) which in the rat can be purified and separated from 1-naphthol-GT (Bock et al., Biochem. Pharmacol. 26, 1097 (1977)) can be assayed in 10 mg liver biopsies. Activated morphine-GT was 0.07 $\pm$ 0.02 μmol/min/ g liver (n=18). GT activities with morphine and 1-naphthol as substrates were correlated in biopsies from 18 patients (r=0.58, p< 0.01). A lack of alternate substrate inhibition was found for the two GTs. The assays may help to elucidate the multiplicity of GT as well as the effects of inducers and pathological factors on the activity of GT in human tissues.

Department of Pharmacology and Toxicology of the University, Kreuzbergring 57, D-3400 Göttingen

47

Effect of Insulin on UDP-Glucuronyltransferase (UDP-GT) Activity and on p-Nitrophenol (pNP) Conjugation Rate in Isolated Perfused Livers from Normal, Fasted, and Diabetic Rats.
P. Bellemann, H. Metzler, and H. Wolburg[*]

This study was designed to further approach the effect of insulin on the conjugation rate of foreign compounds (pNP, 100 μM) in perfused livers from normal, fasted, and diabetic (db) rats. The conjugates (pNP-glucuronide, pNPGA and pNP-sulphate, pNPS) formed during 90 min were estimated after specific enzymatic fission by measuring the liberated pNP at 405 nm. UDP-GT activity was determined by a radioisotopic test (^{14}C-naphthol as substrate) and liver glycogen (l.g.) content was assayed enzymatically.

The amount of conjugates formed and l.g. were significantly reduced in livers from fasted and either alloxan and streptozotocin rats. The pNPGA/pNPS ratio was obviously changed to a preferable sulphation in db livers. The presence of insulin dose-relatedly accelerated the time course of pNPGA and pNPS formation to nearly normal rates. UDP-GT activity, however, was not significantly induced by insulin. Electron micrographes revealed the functional integrity of liver tissue, a depletion of l.g., an increase in SER, but no cell necrosis were detectable.

The results indicate a predominating metabolic pathway for pNP as sulphate in fasted and db rat liver, and l.g. content might influence the conjugate formation. Because of insulin stimulated UDP-GT only slightly with a simultaneously restored pNP conjugation rate, an alteration in the membrane permeability for nutritive substrates by insulin is suggested for the effects reported here.

[*] Pathologisches Institut
Physiologisch-chemisches Institut der Universität, D-7400 Tübingen, Auf dem Schnarrenberg

48

BIOTRANSFORMATION OF 4-DIMETHYLAMINOPHENOL -^{14}C (DMAP) IN RAT LIVER AND ERYTHROCYTES
P. Eyer and H. Kampffmeyer

DMAP rapidly forms ferrihemoglobin and is used for treatment of cyanide poisoning.
Single pass perfusion with modified protein-free Krebs-Henseleit solution showed that 50 per cent of the substrate was removed at prehepatic DMAP of about 0.2 mM. The main route of biotransformation was conjugation. At steady state condition the glucuronide and sulfate formation had an apparent V_{max} of 8 and 1 μmoles per min per g protein and K_m of 500 and 40 μM DMAP, respectively. DMAP-glucuronide was stored by the liver; it was released with a half life of 15 min at a flow rate of 4 ml perfusate per g liver per min.
5 Per cent of the radioactivity was excreted in the bile, essentially as DMAP-glucuronide. Less than 1% of radioactivity was irreversibly bound to liver proteins. Thioethers of DMAP could not be detected in the liver efflux.
The other important path of DMAP biotransformation was demonstrated by addition of human or rat erythrocytes, namely thioether formation with glutathione and SH-groups of hemoglobin. The pattern of DMAP-conjugation was affected depending on the time of prehepatic exposure to erythrocytes, and the species of red cells.

Pharmakologisches Institut der Universität, Nussbaumstrasse 26, D-8000 München 2

49

METABOLISM OF ISOTHIOCYANATES IN RATS   W.H. Mennicke, G. Krumbiegel, and K. Görler

Benzyl, allyl, methyl, ethyl, and butylisothiocyanate occur in plants in the glucosinolate form. When the plant is damaged, these compounds are set free by the enzyme myrosinase. After oral application to rats, the named iso-thiocyanates were excreted renally as mercapturic acids ($R-NH-C-S-CH_2-CH-COOH$; $R=C_6H_5CH_2-$, $CH_2=CH-CH_2-$, CH_3-,
$\quad\quad\quad\quad S \quad\quad HN-COCH_3$

C_2H_5-, C_4H_9-).

Until now, α-naphthyl,ß-naphthyl, and phenylisothiocya-nate have not been found in nature and can only be synthe-tically obtained. After oral application of these com-pounds to rats, the mercapturic acids corresponding to those of the structural equivalent isothiocyanates occu-ring in nature (reaction of the isothiocyanate group with the mercapto group) could not be found neither in the urine nor in the bile. Hitherto, only free α-naphthylamine was clearly identified as a metabolite in the urine and bile after giving α-naphthylisothiocyanate (ANIT). The renal excretion of this metabolite, traced over 96 hours, was 4.4 ± 0.6 % of the applied dose, by a dose of 4 mg ANIT/kg, and 5.5 ± 1.9 %, by a dose of 40 mg ANIT/kg. Biliary excretion, in the time span of 48 hours, was 0.7 ± 0.4% (dose: 4 mg/kg) and 1.5 ± 0.4 % (dose: 40 mg/kg) respec-tively. After giving ß-naphthylisothiocyanate, free ß-naphthylamine and N-acetyl-ß-naphthylamine were identi-fied as metabolites. After administration of phenyliso-thiocyanate, aniline and acetanilide were found, whereby the existence of p-hydroxyacetanilide is probable.

Department of Biochemistry, Dr. Madaus u. Co., D-5000 Cologne 91, Ostmerheimer Str. 198

50

CONJUGATION OF PARACETAMOL DURING TRANSFER ACROSS INTESTINAL MUCOSA OF THE RAT   U. Ehlert, I. Schombert, and H.P. Büch

Isolated jejunal and ileal segments of female Wistar rats were perfused (Fisher and Parsons) with Krebs-Henseleit solution ($37°C$, pH 7,4). Paracetamol (P) was offered at the mucosal side in 50 ml perfusion fluid/segment. P-glucuronide (PG) and P-sulfate (PS) can be measured after high pressure liquid chromatography UV-photo-metrically (250 nm). - PS was not found in the 2-h-absorbate (at least $3 \times 10^{-6}M$ can be de-tected). PG is formed, yet in the jejunum to a considerably higher amount than in the ileum (Tab.). In the jejunum PG formation increases

$[P]$	% of P offered in the 2-h-absorbate					
	jejunum			ileum		
$\times 10^{-3}M$	PG	P	n	PG	P	n
0,66	7,1	3,1	7-14	3,9	4,0	13-14
3,31	3,0	5,3	15	1,1	3,2	10-11
9,93	1,1	6,1	17	0,4	3,2	19-20
33,11	0,09	2,1	13-15	0,02	1,0	13

absolutely more than 2-fold (from 2,35 to 5,20 µM/segment) if concentration of P raises 15-fold (starting at $0,66 \times 10^{-3}M$). Percentage and ab-solute amount of PG are lowest as well in jeju-num as in ileum when concentration of P offered is highest. This indicates that glucuronidation is inhibited by substrate excess.

Department of Pharmacology and Toxicology, University of the Saarland, D-665 Homburg/Saar
Supp. by DFG

51

UV-INDUCED UNSCHEDULED DNA-SYNTHESIS IN DAMAGED SPLE-NIC LYMPHOCYTES OF THE RAT   K. Tempel and R. Hollatz

Unscheduled DNA-synthesis is performed by numerous pro-and eukaryotic cells in response to various nu-cleotoxic influences (see P.C.Hanawalt and R.B.Set-low, ed., Molecular Mechanisms for Repair of DNA, New York, London: Plenum 1975). Since hydroxyurea (HU) has been shown to suppress semiconservative DNA-syn-thesis, it is suggested that the incorporation of a DNA precursor in the presence of HU might be a simple and sensitive-though not specific-test of an impair-ment of nuclear functions. This assumption is con-firmed by the present investigations using unschedu-led ($10^{-2}M$ HU) UV-stimulated ^3H-thymidine (^3H-TdR, methyl-^3H-thymidine, 40-60 Ci/mmol) incorporation in vitro into splenic lymphocytes (about 2×10^7 cells per ml Hank's solution) of rats after total-body X-irradiation (TBI) and/or i.p. injection of 2,4,6-tri-ethyleneimino-s-triazine (TEM). - The results may be summarized as follows: 1. Unscheduled TdR-^3H incorpo-ration into splenic lymphocytes of rats decreased im-mediately after TBI (3-1000 rad) in a dose-dependent manner. - 2. Maximum effects could be obtained with-in 4-8 hours after exposure to the $DL_{50/30}$ of TBI. - 3. A TBI-dose of 6,25 rad was demonstrable ($p<0,01$).-4. Following a sublethal TBI (250 rad), regeneration of the repair activity has taken about 4-6 weeks. - 5. Analogous effects have been shown using TEM; the combination of TBI and TEM resulted in additive or even potentiating interactions. - Different mechanisms should be regarded: With respect to early postirra-diation periods, expansion of the TdR-pool, disturban-ces of the nuclear energy metabolism, and/or damage of the DNA-matrix might be implicated. Regarding la-ter posttreatment periods, one cannot exclude popula-tion changes within the splenic cellularity.

Institut für Pharmakologie,Toxikologie und Pharmazie, FB Tiermedizin, Universität München, Königinstr. 16

52

STUDY OF INTOXICATIONS WITH DIETHYLPENTENAMIDE AND STRUCTURE ELUCIDATION OF ITS METABOLITES BY GC-MS-TECHNIQUE   W. Ehrenthal, and K. Pfleger

Diethylpentenamide (DPA) is a hypnotic which is sold with-out prescription in W-Germany since 1975. Suicides with this drug have greatly increased in the past two years and will further increase when the bromoureides are under prescription. Measurement of the blood concentration of DPA is necessary for prognosis and therapy. Under the conditions of intensive medicine care there is no danger for the patient's life up to a drug concentration of 5 mg/100 ml blood. With higher concentration of DPA and additional clinical risks detoxication by haemoperfusion (Haemocol) may be helpful. Its clearance for DPA (118.2 $\pm$ 4.1 ml/min, n = 11) is the same as for Carbromal (110.4 $\pm$ 3.9, n = 43). The half life of DPA in blood considering low concentrations is 7.7 h. However, in severe poisoned patients it will be longer. Drug metabolism is the main route for elimination and the amount of the unchanged drug in the urine extract is very little compaired with the metabolites. Besides 3.3-diethyl-5-hydroxymethyl-tetra-hydro-2-furanone, which is already known in literature,
   3.3-diethyl-tetrahydro-2-furanone-5-carboxylic acid,
   3.3-diethyl-2-pyrrolidone-5-carboxylic acid,
   3.3-diethyl-5-hydroxymethyl-2-pyrrolidone, and
   2.2-diethyl-4-keto-valeriamylamide
have been found. The structures of these new metabolites have been elucidated by GC-MS-measurements with low and high resolution. As a substance which is structure - related to allyl-isopropyl-acetylcarbamide (Sedormid) DPA may as well provoke porphyria. Indeed porphyria was observed in one patient and it must be mentioned that in this case the coma due to overdose of DPA was largely intensified.

Department of Pharmacology and Toxicology, University of the Saarland, D-665 Homburg/Saar

53

MASS FRAGMENTOGRAPHIC STUDY OF THE TIME COURSE OF DIFFE-
RENT DRUGS WITH RESPECT TO THE PLASMA-SALIVARY DISTRIBU-
TION COEFFICIENT IN MAN
R. Eckard, R. Ening, and W. Ening

After oral application of diphenhydramine (I), 2,2-diethyl-
allyl-acetamide (II), carbromal (III) and paracetamol (IV)
in man, equilibration of drug concentrations between blood
plasma and resting saliva was measured up to 24 hrs. The
drug concentrations were determined by means of gaschroma-
tographic-mass fragmentographic methods using single-ion-
detection (SID) at characteristic m/e values of these compounds (m/e 165 (I), m/e 126 (II), m/e 167 (III) and m/e
1o9 (IV) after methylation by means of diazomethane).
Despite of the different pharmacokinetic behaviour and the
different physicochemical properties, all investigated
drugs revealed a nearly constant plasma-salivary distribution coefficient within 24 hrs. The obtained mean plasma-
saliva ratios were o.26 $\pm$ o.o2 (I), o.96 $\pm$ o.o4 (II),
1.24 $\pm$ o.o3 and o.93 $\pm$ o.o4 (IV) respectively. These
ratios seem to be specific for each drug depending on
their pK-values, lipophilic characters and plasma protein
binding abilities; they are obviously unaffected by changes
of plasma drug concentrations. Both neutral drugs (III and
IV) as well as weak acids as the phenolic drug paracetamol
show distribution coefficient values near one, whereas the
basic antihistamine I (pK$_a$ = 8.8) is excreted in remarkable
higher salivary concentrations according to the pH-gradient
theory, due to the difference of pH-values between saliva
and plasma.

Thus, saliva indicates to be a readily available and reliable body fluid in drug abuse monitoring.

Institute of Pharmacology and Toxicology, University of
Münster, Westring 12, D-44oo Münster

54

THE EFFECT OF 4-DIMETHYLAMINOPHENOL ON
ACID-BASE BALANCE, LACTATE, PYRUVATE,
LOCAL CEREBRAL BLOOD FLOW AND BRAIN TEM-
PERATURE OF DOGS AFTER ACUTE CYANIDE
POISONING R. Klimmek, C. Roddewig, and N. Weger

Male beagles were anesthetized with chloralose (50 mg/
kg i.v.). Local cerebral blood flow (CBF) was determined with thermocouples in the cingulum region of the
right hemisphere, and brain temperature in the left
hemisphere. Arterial pO_2, pCO_2, and pH were
measured continuously with electrodes. Hemoglobin,
lactate, and pyruvate were determined at constant time
intervals. The dogs were poisoned with KCN, 4 mg/kg
i.v., and 1 min later they were treated with 4-dimethyl-
aminophenol (DMAP), 3.25 mg/kg i.v.
Cyanide induced hyperventilation for 30 sec, followed
by respiratory arrest. Then, respiratory minute volume
increased by 70% within 10 min and remained elevated
at a lower level. Hemoglobin concentration rose by
24% within 10 min and then returned to normal. PO_2
increased by 200 mmHg within 3 min and reached
100 mmHg within another 3 min. After decreasing by
8 mmHg within 2 min, pCO_2 tended to increase within a
few minutes while pH was falling. Base-excess diminished by 6 meq/l and remained lowered to the same
extent. The lactate-pyruvate quotient fell from 24 to
19.6 within 5 min and then increased to 30. Local ther-
mic transport (CBF) increased by 70% and then decreased
rapidly to nearly control values. Brain temperature
diminished by 0.37^{o}C within 15 min, the fall being retarded by a transient increase of 0.16^{o}C. Then the
temperature tended to increase.

Pharmakologisches Institut der Universität München,
D-8000 München 2, Nussbaumstrasse 26

55

COMBINED EFFECTS: ACUTE TOXICITY OF LOCAL ANESTHETICS IN
BINARY AND TERNARY MIXTURES AMONG THEMSELVES OR WITH
EPINEPHRINE IN ISOBOLOGRAPHIC PRESENTATION J. Hamacher
and M. Kuhn

The local anesthetics: Procaine (NOVOCAIN), tetracaine
(PANTOCAIN), lidocaine (XYLOCAIN), butanilicaine (HOSTA-
CAIN), mepivacaine (SCANDICAIN), tolycaine (BAYCAIN) and
carticaine (ULTRACAIN) were investigated for their acute
intravenous toxicity in mice, alone and in various binary
or ternary mixtures among themselves or with epinephrine
as vasoconstrictor.

The experimental results are assembled for graphic presentation in form of multiple isobolograms(FRASER, LOEWE)
to indicate whether the combined effects are equal to,
or greater or less than, those expected by simple addition.

From altogether 12o different combinations of theoretical
equal toxicity showed 57 (47,5 per cent) an increase, 31
(25,8 per cent) a decrease but only 32 (26,7 per cent) an
additive behaviour.

From 63 different binary local anesthetics mixtures of
theoretical equal toxicity showed 31 an increase, 14 a
decrease and 18 an additive behaviour.

From 42 different binary local anesthetic epinephrine
mixtures of theoretical equal toxicity showed 18 an increase, 16 a decrease but only 8 an additive behaviour.

From 15 different ternary local anesthetics epinephrine
mixtures of theoretical equal toxicity showed 8 an increase, 1 a decrease and 6 an additive behaviour.

These results may warn of thoughtless combining of local
anesthetics among themselves in medical use.

Prof.Dr.med. J.Hamacher, Pharmakologisches Institut der
Universität, 5ooo Köln 41, Gleueler Str. 24

56

INVESTIGATION ON THE KINETIC PROPERTIES OF A CARRIER-
BOUND ACETYLCHOLINESTERASE (E.C.3.1.1.7) IN A
COLUMN   C. Alsen, S. Bhattacharya and P. Valentin
Acetylcholinesterase (AChE)(E.C.3.1.1.7) covalently bound
to polymaleinic anhydride was found to be one of the best immo-
bilized AChE preparations retaining most of the characteristics of
the free enzyme. The present study was undertaken in order to
investigate its properties in a Celite 545, (20-45 u) column
(0.6 cm x 1.75 cm; total bed vol.-0.5 ml void vol.-0.36 ml) at
optimum conditions with respect to temp. (30°C) and pH (7.8).
1. An usual bell shaped pS activity curve was obtained at all flow
rates studied, the optimum concentration lying between 2×10^{-3}M -
4×10^{-3}M Acetylthiocholine. 2. Percentage of substrate hydrolysed
as a function of flow rate and initial substrate concentration
showed inverse relationships. 3. The apparent Km calculated at
different flow rates was always found to be greater (1×10^{-2}M -
1×10^{-3}M) than that obtained in the stirred suspension (1.92 x
10^{-4}M). 4. Inhibition of the column by carbaryl, paraoxon and
combination of carbaryl and paraoxon were studied at a flow rate
of 0.8 ml/min. The K_2 value for paraoxon (1.98×10^5 xM^{-1} xmin^{-1})
was slightly lower than that in the stirred suspension (3×10^5
xM^{-1} xmin^{-1}). The rate of inhibition by carbaryl (1×10^{-6}M,
1×10^{-7}M) and a combination of paraoxon (2×10^{-7}M) and
carbaryl (1×10^{-6}M) of the AChE in the column preparation was
also found to be slower than that determined by the pH-stat method.
Preliminary observations suggest the practical applicability of this
preparation to the detection of AChE inhibitors in water samples.

Untersuchungsstelle für Umwelttoxikologie des Landes Schleswig-
Holstein, D 23 Kiel, Fleckenstrasse

57

STUDIES ON THE ACTION OF CHLORAMPHENICOL AND ITS ANALOGS ON 55S, 70S, and 80S RIBOSOMES: B. Ulbrich & W. Czempiel

Ribosomes from bacteria, eucaryotes (cytoplasm), and mitochondria (higher animals) are typified by their different S-values: 70S, 80S, 55S. The 70S and 80S categories exhibit relatively uniform chemical and physical properties, whereas mitochondrial ribosomes display many individual species with great structural diversity. Chemotherapeutic agents which inhibit defined steps of translation have been used to gain insight into the mechanism of protein synthesis or on the relationship between mitochondrial and non-mitochondrial ribosomes. To investigate differences in the mode of action of chloramphenicol (CAP) and its analogs on the 3 types of ribosomes, the following experiments were performed: 1) CAP and its analogs in similar concentrations ($\leq$15 µg/ml) inhibit protein synthesis of mitochondria and bacteria but not of 80S ribosomes. 2) ^{14}C-CAP in equilibrium dialysis experiments binds to E.coli and mitochondrial but not to 80S ribosomes. The number of binding sites for the 2 types of ribosomes is 2. Competition and affinity labeling experiments will have to show whether differences exist in the binding sites, affinity of CAP compared to analogs, and the localization of this site. 3) Peptidyl-transferase activity is inhibited in 70S and 55S ribosomes over 75% at 0.5 mM CAP; 80S ribosomes are insensitive. 4) Poly-U directed poly-phe synthesis is partially inhibited by CAP in E.coli and mitochondrial but not in 80S ribosomes. 5) 2-Dimensional separation by polyacrylamide gel electrophoresis of the proteins of 70S, 55S, and 80S ribosomes reveals different patterns and numbers of protein spots for all 3 types. - Our data support the idea that therapeutic side-effects of CAP and its analogs exerted by inhibition of protein synthesis are caused only at the mitochondrial ribosomal level. It is conceivable that CAP in mitochondria like in bacteria acts by inhibition of peptidyl-transferase. -   Supported by DFG grants (Sfb 29). Institut für Toxikologie und Embryonal-Pharmakologie, Freie Universität Berlin, Garystr. 9, 1 Berlin 33

58

DIAPLACENTAL TRANSFER OF THIAMPHENICOL (TAP) IN PREGNANT RATS DURING LATE ORGANOGENESIS   R. Bass and I. Schütte

The application of chemotherapeutic agents during organogenesis which in mammals specifically interfere with mitochondrial biogenesis and function leads to impaired embryonal development. Whereas lower doses of chloramphenicol (CAP) or TAP lead to reversible inhibition of both mitochondrial and embryonal development, higher doses lead to embryolethality via mitochondrial impairment (D. Oerter & R. Bass, Naunyn-Schmiedeberg's Arch. Pharmacol. 290, 175, 1975; R. Bass & D. Oerter, ibid. 296, 191, 1977). The effects were also dependent on time and duration of treatment. CAP in the rat is very rapidly eliminated as glucuronide with a serum half-life of about 25 min (J. Alvin & B.N. Dixit, Biochem. Pharmacol. 23, 139, 1974). 1 g/kg CAP infused i.v. for 24 h (day 12 of gestation) yields levels in maternal serum and fetal tissues of about 20 µg per ml or g, and reversibly inhibits mitochondrial protein synthesis and embryonal development. 125 mg TAP/kg (day 10 and 11), or 80 mg/kg (days 10-13) strongly inhibit mitochondrial biosynthesis and lead to embryolethality. As a first prerequisite to extrapolate the experimental findings to the human situation the pharmacokinetic behaviour of TAP in rats was studied after a single s.c. injection on day 12.

TABLE:	Time after Appl.:	2-3 h	6 h	12 h	24 h
100 mg/kg	Maternal Serum	14.5	3.2	0.68	0.18
	Embryo	6.8	2.7	0.69	0.18
50 mg/kg	Maternal Serum	5.0	0.6	data are given	
	Embryo	3.8	0.6	as µg per ml or g	

In man 7-15 mg TAP/kg given 3 times daily are used for treatment of bacterial infections yielding peak serum concentrations of 10-20 µg/ml (half-life about 2 h). When TAP in humans also freely crosses the placental barrier and if mitochondrial biosynthesis is equally sensitive to TAP as in the rat embryo, one could conclude that prolonged exposure to the drug is harmful to human embryos.
Supported by DFG grants, Institut für Toxikologie & Embryonal-Pharmakologie, Freie Universität, Garystr.9, 1 Berlin 33

59

DIAPLACENTAL TRANSFER AND FETAL DISTRIBUTION OF THIAMPHENICOL IN EARLY HUMAN PREGNANCY H. Nau, F. Welsch & H.Egger

A single dose of 500 mg thiamphenicol (TAP) was given to 30 women at various times prior to interruption of pregnancy for social and/or medical reasons during the first trimester (curettage, hysterotomy, or prostaglandin induction). Concentrations of TAP were then determined in maternal serum, placental, and fetal tissues by a gas chromatographic method using electron capture detection. Similar, but sometimes significantly higher, concentrations of TAP were found in placental and fetal tissues as compared to maternal serum (data expressed as µg/ml or µg/g).

Time after Application	Maternal Serum	Placenta	Fetal Organs			
			Muscle	Liver	Kidney	Brain
2.5 h	4.4	6.4	4.5		4.5	2.7
4 h	3.6	21	6.3	3.4	3.0	1.6
10 h	0.74		0.37	2.1	1.9	1.6
20 h	0.2	0.21	0.16	0.32	0.27	0.21

Uptake of TAP (10 µg/ml of Hank's balanced salt solution) *in vitro* into free-hand dissected fragments of immature and term placentas was measured following incubation that lasted from 5 to 120 min. Concentrations were determined in the intracellular space by deducting TAP present in extracellular space as determined with ^{14}C-inulin. Both tissues were able to accumulate the drug.
Since TAP reaches the human fetus during early human pregnancy at concentrations at least similar to maternal serum concentrations, one might conclude that this drug is a useful chemotherapeutic for the treatment of fetal infections. However, if human fetal mitochondria prove equally susceptible to those from rat embryos, a prolonged exposure to TAP is expected to be harmful to the human embryo. The significance of placental accumulation of TAP requires further investigations.
Supported by DFG grants (Sfb 29), Institut für Toxikologie und Embryonal-Pharmakologie, Freie Universität Berlin, Garystr. 9, D-1000 Berlin 33, West-Germany.

60

ACTIVITIES OF THE UNSPECIFIC HYDROXYLASES, EPOXIDE HYDRASE AND GLUTATHIONE S-TRANSFERASE IN HUMAN LIVER MICROSOMES AND CYTOSOL DURING RIFAMPICIN TREATMENT. Fleischmann, R., J. Lorenz, and H. U. Schmassmann

In previous studies we could demonstrate that the amount of cytochrome P-450 in human liver homogenate increases 3- to 4-fold if patients are treated with rifampicin (Drug Metab. Dispos. 1, 224, 1973). The rate of drug oxidation measured as O-demethylation of p-nitroanisole, N-demethylation of aminopyrine in vitro and the excretion of the novaminsulfonum metabolite 4-aminoantipyrine in vivo was only slightly increased. In contrast, Bolt et al. measured a 5-fold enhanced oxidation rate of oestradiol and ethinyl-oestradiol at C-2 position of the aromatic ring in liver microsomes of patients treated with rifampicin (Europ. J. Clin. Pharmacol. 8, 301, 1975). However, rifampicin was not able to induce these parameters in experiments with mice, rats and guinea pigs (unpubl.). It was assumed that rifampicin treatment induces a special form of cyt. P-450. In order to receive more reliable results, microsomes from human liver needle biopsy material were prepared and the activities of cyt.-c-reductase, aryl hydrocarbon hydroxylase (fluorometrically), 7-ethoxycoumarin-O-dealkylase (with and without inhibitors), and the epoxide hydratase measured. The activity of glutathione S-transferase was determined in the 100 000 x g supernatant of the same preparations. In 12 control patients we found a small variation in the activities of microsomal enzymes (standard deviation not higher than 20 %). A decrease could be detected in patients with hepatitis and biliary diseases. During rifampicin treatment (10 mg/kg daily) we found a 10- to 15-fold increase of aryl hydrocarbon hydroxylase activity from 45.5 $\pm$ 10.8 to 491.4 $\pm$ 122.4 FU per mg microsomal protein, but only a doubling of the O-dealkylation rate of 7-ethoxycoumarin. However, naphthoflavone (10^{-5} M) did not inhibit the O-dealkylation as in liver microsomes of untreated patients, presenting further evidence for an unusual type of cyt. P-450 induced by rifampicin.
Dr. R. Fleischmann, Medizinische Universitätsklinik, Auf dem Schnarrenberg, D-7400 Tübingen

61

THE INFLUENCE OF AGE ON HEAVY-METAL-CONCENTRATIONS IN HUMAN TISSUE   P.Weigert and H.Fischer

Samples of tissue taken from the liver, kidneys and the brain of persons who in most of the cases died suddenly or by lethal accident, have been analyzed by means of atomicabsorption-spectrometry (H.Fischer, P.Weigert Öff.Gesundh.-Wesen 37,732-737 (1975) and 39, 269-278 (1977)). The object of the analysis were the respective contents of lead (Pb), cadmium (Cd), mercury (Hg), copper (Cu), manganese (Mn) and zinc (Zn). After classification into age groups, the influence of age on the heavy-metal content in the various organs was probed into by means of correlation analyses. No dependence was found with Mn, Zn and, especially, Hg, the reason for this being the relatively short biological half-value period of those metals. A heavy concentration of Cu was found in the liver of very young persons only (up to one year old), further aging being of no consequence to the Cu content. The concentration of Pb in the liver, however, increases markedly with age (R= 0,65; P< 0,02). Striking correlations were found for Cd in the brain and liver (R= 0,85; P< 0,001), whereas, due to the largely scattered pattern of measured values, this effect did not appear as marked in the kidneys (R= 0,70; P< 0,01).

Veterinär-Untersuchungsstelle der Bundeswehr VI
Dachauer Str. 128, 8000 München 19

62

CADMIUM CONTENT OF MUSHROOMS   R. Seeger

The cadmium content of 402 species of wild mushrooms, either edible or poisonous, was determined by flameless atomic absorption spectroscopy. Of each species several samples - altogether 1049 - of different origin were tested, if possible. The mushrooms were collected in various European countries, mainly in southern Germany, 1967 to 1977.
The cadmium content was between < 0.1 and 120 mg/kg dry weight, equivalent to < 0.01 and 10.8 mg/kg fresh weight. Low cadmium levels were predominant:

mg cadmium/kg dry weight	% of samples
< 2	67.7
2- 5	18.6
5-10	5.5
10-20	4.0
20-50	2.5
> 50	1.7

The cadmium content was clearly species-dependent, and to a lesser extent genus-dependent. Samples containing more than 10 mg/kg dry weight occurred in 41 species, among these were 9 Tricholomataceae, 10 Agaricaceae, 11 Cortinariaceae, 3 Amanitas, and 4 Russula species. Samples containing more than 50 mg/kg dry weight were found in Agaricus (A.) augustus, A. perrarus, A. silvicola, A. macrosporus, A. maleolens, and Inocybe bongardii.
In single fruit-bodies the lowest cadmium content was found in the stem, whereas the highest content was found in the gills and tubes. Cadmium content of the gills was at most 5 times the amount present in the fleshy part of the cap.
In cadmium-rich mushrooms a marked concentration had occurred as compared with the cadmium content of the soil.

Supported by the Deutsche Forschungsgemeinschaft

Institut für Pharmakologie und Toxikologie der Universität
Versbacher Landstrasse 9, D-8700 Würzburg

63

INFLUENCE OF LOW CADMIUM-DOSAGES IN SUBACUTE EXPERIMENTS ON THE DRUG METABOLISM ON MICE.
J.Abel, H.Dieter, H.Menzel, and F.K.Ohnesorge

Almost nothing is known of the actions of subacute or chronic exposure to Cadmium on liver enzymes and its interactions with drug metabolism. Therefore, male mice were i.p. dosed with 0; 0,003; 0,01; 0,03; 0,1 and 0,3mg Cd^{++}/kg b.w. x day (as $CdCl_2$) for 20 consecutive days. From day 22. to 26. they were treated with Phenobarbital (50mg/kgxday). Controls received NaCl. On day 27. the Hexobarbital-sleeping time was measured and the mice were killed on day 28. - The determination of several drug metabolizing enzymes in liver microsomes and cytosol revealed a strong influence of low doses of Cd, especially in Phenobarbital (PhB)-induced mice. - There was a prolongation of the sleeping time by 0,03mg Cd in PhB-free and PhB-treated mice. Cytochrom-P-450 and the activity of the N-Demethylase corresponded roughly to the sleeping time. - The activity of the mixed-functional Oxidase (Substr. Benzpyrene) was increased (0,3-0,01mg; PhB-ind.), whereas the activity of the Epoxide-Hydratase was not influenced by Cd. - The Glutathion-Aralkyl-Transferase activity showed an inhibition in PhB-free as well as in PhB-treated mice (0,3-0,01mg). The Glutathion-S-Epoxid-Transferase was inhibited by 0,3mg Cd (PhB-free and PhB-ind.) and was increased in PhB-treated mice by lower Cd-doses (0,1-0,01mg). Accordingly, the Glutathion content of the liver was affected only by 0,3mg Cd. - Our results point to a possible cocarcinogenic action of Cadmium and demonstrate new aspects on the evaluation of Cadmium risks.

Department of Toxicology, University of Düsseldorf,
D-4000 Düsseldorf, Moorenstr. 5

64

IN VIVO APPLICATION OF COBALT MODIFIES ACTIVITY PATTERNS OF MICROSOMAL MONOOXYGENASE   W. Legrum

Cobaltous chloride has been shown to reduce the concentration of microsomal cytochrome P 450 in rats (Tephly & Hibbeln, BBRC 42, 589, 1971). In non-induced C57BL/6J mice the cytochrome P 450 concentration was decreased to about 60 % of the original value after two daily s.c. applications of 40 mg/kg $CoCl_2$. In PB or MC induced animals this decrase is not as marked.

The deethylation of 7-ethoxycoumarin was studied in vitro in relation to time and dosage of cobalt pretreatment of control and PB-induced animals, whereby activity is expressed in relation to cytochrome P 450. In controls cobalt produces after two days a fourfold increase in 7-hydroxycoumarin formation while in PB-induced animals this increase is only 2.5 fold. In contrast, no activity increase was observed with ethoxyresorufin as substrate for dealkylation.

Inhibition of 7-ethoxycoumarin deethylation by metyrapone results in a strong shift of the dose-effect-curve to lower inhibitor concentrations by cobalt pretreatment. Cobalt microsomes are fifty times more sensitive than controls. A similar effect is seen after PB pretreatment of the mice. This is taken as evidence for a cobalt-induced transformation of cytochrome P 450 to a PB-like variety with respect to metyrapone inhibition. Ethoxyresorufin deethylation is inhibited by metyrapone in a two step mode resulting in a long plateau in the dose-response-curve. Inflection points of both parts of the inhibition curve are very distinct, the difference between the respective metyrapone concentrations being 10 000 fold.

It is concluded that cobalt pretreatment modifies the constitutive composition of microsomal cytochrome(s) in a way similar to PB and produces characteristic inhibition patterns with different substrates.

This work was supported by the Deutsche Forschungsgemeinschaft.

Department of Pharmacology and Toxicology, University of Marburg, Lahnberge, D-3550 Marburg, Germany

65

BEHAVIOURAL DEVIATIONS IN RATS CHRONICALLY EX-
POSED TO LEAD AT THE ACCEPTED NO-EFFECT LEVEL.

E. Groß-Selbeck

Male Wistar rats after weaning were fed a daily
diet containing 1g/kg food for a period of 20
weeks until the lead level reached 21-24 μg/100
ml blood. This blood-lead level is considered to
be harmless to man.

The general behaviour in the open-field task was
tested with the following parameters: locomotion
(central fields entered, peripheral fields entered), local movement (rearing and grooming behaviour), emotionality (defecation). The conditioned instrumental behaviour was tested in the
Skinner box in a series of increasingly difficult
programmes.

The open-field behaviour showed no overt neuro-
logical impairment of the rats. Similarly, no effects in preliminary instrumental training could
be observed. However, differences between controls and treated animals became evident with increasing difficulty of the programmes, such as a
sequence of differential reinforcements of high
rates and a series of opposite conditioning tasks
(differential reinforcement of low rates, fixed
interval reinforcement).

It is concluded from these experiments that lead
exposure to man at doses which presently are suggested to be innocuous may induce subclinical
functional changes of the central nervous system
(CNS). Such effects may become evident when sensitive behavioural tests are performed.

Dept. of Toxicology, Gesellschaft für Strahlen-
u. Umweltforschung, D-8042 Neuherberg.

66

OXIDATION OF ELEMENTAL MERCURY BY RED-CELL
ENZYMES. S. Halbach.

The incorporation of atomic Hg in erythrocytes
can be inhibited by ethanol or stimulated by
H_2O_2 (F.Nielsen-Kudsk, Arch.Pharmacol.Toxicol.
27, 161, 1969), and three mechanisms are considered for the oxidation of the metal: formation of GSH radicals by glutathione-peroxidase
(GSH-Px), nascent O_2 from the catalatic break-
down of H_2O_2 or the peroxidatic reaction of catalase complex I. To select among these, genetically different erythrocytes with various
enzyme activities had been used.
Catalase activity was high in human, medium in
normal-mouse (Cs-a), low in acatalasemic-mouse
(Cs-b) and absent in duck erythrocytes. GSH-Px
activity was low in human, medium in duck and
high in Cs-a and Cs-b cells. The Hg uptake increased from 25 to 770 ng/(mg Hb x 45 min) in
human and from 9 to 151 in Cs-a cells with increasing H_2O_2 infusion rates, which nevertheless excluded the evolution of O_2. No Hg uptake
at all was found in Cs-b and duck erythrocytes.
In presence of 60 mM 3-amino-1,2,4-triazole the
inhibition of Hg oxidation in human red cells
was closely correlated to the inactivation of
catalase. In Cs-a cells the inhibition of GSH-
Px by 1 mM iodoactate raised the Hg uptake over
that of controls. The peroxidatic reaction with
complex I is likely to be the main factor for
the biological oxidation of Hg in erythrocytes.

Abtlg. Pharmakologie, Gesellschaft für Strahlen-
und Umweltforschung, D-8042 Neuherberg.

67

SODIUM-2,3-DIMERCAPTOPROPANESULFONATE: PHARMACO-
KINETIC DATA AND THERAPY OF MERCURY POISONING

B. Gabard

The water-soluble derivative of BAL, Sodium-2,3-
dimercaptopropanesulfonate (DMPS) has shown very good
results in improving the urinary elimination of Hg in
cases of poisoning with inorganic as well as with
organic Hg compounds (B. Gabard, Arch. Toxicol., 35,
15, 1976 and Toxicol. Appl. Pharmacol., 38, 415,1976).
For the first time, pharmacokinetic data were
obtained in the rat using 1,3-^{14}C-labeled DMPS. Over
a wide dose range (0.1-1.0 mmol/kg), the distribution
does not depend on the dose. The highest concentrations are found immediately after injection in the
kidneys (7.4±0.04 % of the dose/g wet weight) and in
plasma (2.3±0.02 %/ml), the lowest in the brain
(0.06±0.04 %/g). The excretion is very rapid (T1/2 =
19 min) and follows a monoexponential curve in plasma
and in most of the organs during the first hour after
the injection. 80-90 % of the dose are excreted
within the first 6 hours. The plasma clearance of
DMPS equals the glomerular filtration rate of the rat
as measured under steady-state conditions. The apparent volume of distribution of the radioactivity after
an i.v. injection is equivalent to the volume of the
extracellular water. After oral administration 30-40%
are absorbed from the gut. The results of the pharmacokinetic analysis raise the question how an intracellularly deposited metal is removed by an extracellular chelating agent. Furthermore, they explain
the lack of side-effects during treatment of heavy-
metal poisoning with DMPS and make the drug especially suited for chronic poisoning cases.

Institut für Genetik und für Toxikologie von
Spaltstoffen, Kernforschungszentrum Karlsruhe,
Postfach 3640, D-7500 Karlsruhe 1

68

INHIBITORY EFFECT OF CHLORO(TRIETHYLPHOSPHINE)-
GOLD ON RAT PAW EDEMA   L.P.Anda[+]and K.Kasperek[++]

We studied resorption and deposition of the gold
salt in the organs of male W-rats and the effect
on the development of paw edemas experimentally
induced by carrageenin, dextran and kaolin. We
administered p.o. 8.75 mg gold salt = 5.0 mg
metallic gold/kg rat weight daily for seven days.
The gold salt was suspended in tragant. Control
animals were either untreated, or received the
inflammation agent, or else received only 3.0 ml
physiol. saline p.o. On the 8th day, carrageenin,
dextran or kaolin were injected into the l. hind
paw. In a part of the control animals, saline was
injected into the l.hind paw;another part remained
untreated. Two hours after onset of inflammation
the rats were killed and paws and organs examined.
Wt.differences between inflamed and non-inflamed
paws denoted intensity of edema development. The
gold content of paws and organs was measured by
neutron activation analysis (at the Medical Inst.
of the nuclear research station at Jülich). The
findings were: orally administered gold salt was
resorbed during treatment lasting 7 days. The
gold content of the inflamed paws in the groups
given carrageenin, dextran and kaolin was higher
than in the non-inflamed paws of the same groups
(mean values: 2.04 x 10^{-4} g compared to 0.844 x
10^{-4} g). Unlike in controls, edema development
was inhibited by an average of 56.8% (p=0.006).
EM and biochemical studies indicate that the
metallic gold is taken up by the cell and inhibits some of the processes typical for inflammation.

[+] Pharmakologisches Inst.d.Universität, D-53 Bonn
    Federal Republic of Germany.
[++]KFA Jülich GmbH, D-517 Jülich, Postfach 1913,
    Institut für Medizin.

69

Studies on the phalloidin recognizing structure of the liver cell surface. E. Petzinger, M. Frimmer.

Phalloidin, one of the cyclopeptides of Amanita phalloides is exlusively toxic for intact hepatocytes. The specificity of the toxin seems to be related to the recognition by the surface of liver cells, but not to the final reaction with the microsceleton on the inside of the plasma membrane. The phalloidin response (PhR) of isolated hepatocytes is reversibly inhibited by low concentrations of trypsin (Frimmer et al., Naunyn-Schmiedeberg's Arch. Pharmacol. 300, 163-171, 1977) and of phospholipase A (Petzinger et al., Naunyn-Schmiedeberg's Arch. Pharmacol. in press, 1978), indicating that both protein and lipid structures are involved in the uptake of phalloidin. Further studies with chemical agents (protein reagents, crosslinking agents) give additional evidence for the role of a membranal protein in recognition and uptake of phalloidin: Glutardialdehyde blocks the PhR at concentrations below 0.01%. Diisothiocyano-stilbene-disulfonic acid (DIDS) and its dihydroderivative (H$_2$-DIDS) inhibit the PhR in a concentration dependent manner without marked penetration into the cells. The degree of inhibition is related to the concentration of H$_2$-DIDS irreversibly bound to hepatocytes. 1-anilino-8-naphthalene sulfonate (ANS) is also a potent inhibitor, but its effect is partially reversible. Both DIDS and ANS are known to inhibit the anionic transport in red cells. Therefore their activity on the uptake of bile acids by isolated hepatocytes was tested: DIDS inhibited the inward transport of glycolic acid in a non competitive manner. These findings stimulate speculations concerning a possible relationship of the uptake of phalloidin to the inward transport of bile acids.

Dept. Pharmacol. Toxicol., University Giessen, Frankfurter Str. 107, D-6300 Giessen

70

ISOLATION AND CHARACTERIZATION OF CONTRAKTILE PROTEINS FROM PHALLOIDIN INSENSITIVE AS-30D ASCITES HEPATOMA CELLS. E. Grundmann.

Phalloidin, a toxic bicyclic heptapeptide from Amanita phalloides acts on the formation of filamentous structures in the membrane fraction of rat liver (A.M. Lengsfeld et al., Proc. Nat. Acad. Sci. USA 71, 2803, 1974). In vitro phalloidin induces polymerization of muscle G-actin to fibrils (Ph-actin). However, in contrast to muscle F-actin, Ph-actin is resistant against 0.6 M KI (I. Löw et al., FEBS LETTERS 44, 340, 1974).
AS-30D ascites hepatoma cells are insensitive to phalloidin. To elucidate the reason of this insensitivity contractile proteins were isolated from this cell type following the method of M. Clarke et al. (J. Mol. Biol. 86, 209, 1974). A mysoin-like protein of hepatoma cells exhibits a Ca^{2+}ATPase activity of 30 nmol mg^{-1} min^{-1}. Its mol. wt is about 200.000 daltons. An actin-like protein migrates with a mobility corresponding to 43.000 daltons and forms paracrystals in the presence of Mg^{2+} as shown by electron microscopy. In vitro G-actin from hepatoma cells interacts with phalloidin in the same way as muscle G-actin, e.g. inducing polymerization to Ph-actin and partial resistance against 0.6 M KI.
The above results confirm the conclusion that the quantity and reactivity of contractile proteins in hepatoma cells cannot be the cause of the insensitivity against phalloidin. Other investigations suggest that the phalloidin response of normal liver cells needs a specific uptake of the toxin.

Dept. Pharmacol. and Toxicol. University of Giessen Frankfurter Straße 107, D-6300 Giessen-Lahn

71

TOXICOLOGICAL STUDIES ON GYROMITRIN, A POISONOUS COMPOUND IN FALSE MORELS U. Greeff, J. Kremer

Gyromitrin was found as a toxic compound in the false morel Gyromitra esculenta (P.H. List & P. Luft, Arch. Pharm. 301, 384, 1968). The clinical symptoms are similar to that of Amanita phalloides. Systematic investigations with animals have not yet been described.

After application of 200 mg/kg (p.o.) gyromitrin (about 80% of LD$_{50}$) a time dependent decrease of cytochrome P 450 was found in rat liver microsomes. The maximal decrease to about 50 - 60% of the control was observed about 8 h after application, a normalization after 48 h. The inhibition of cyt. P 450 mediated metabolism of aminopyrine, p-nitroanisole, hexobarbitone corresponds to the decrease of cytochrome P 450. The specific activity of cytochrome P 450 remains unchanged. Experiments in vitro with rat liver microsomes show that the influence of gyromitrin (5×10^{-4}M) causes an increased lipid peroxidation. The formation of malondialdehyde increases to about 200% of the control, while the consumption of oxygen rises up to about 160%. This suggests an attack on the endoplasmatic membrane, but not an interference with the oxygenase system.

Furthermore, an intense diuresis was observed after application of gyromitrin, whereby the increased elimination of chloride and potassium is parallel to the increased volume (160 - 200% of the control). In contrast to these results the elimination of sodium increases to about 600%. The evident deficit of chloride is probably compensated for by an enhanced elimination of bicarbonate, which is shown by the alkaline pH of urine. The values of urea and creatinine in serum do not differ from standards in a period of 72 h after application. Diuresis is normalized 144 h after application of gyromitrin.

Institute of Pharmacology and Toxicology, University of Marburg, Lahnberge, D-3550 Marburg/Lahn.

72

THE INFLUENCE OF FASTING ON THE ACTIVITY OF SOME HEPATOTOXIC AGENTS E. Dost

The hepatotoxic effects of 8 compounds were investigated in normally fed mice on the one and in 24-hours fasted mice on the other hand. The extent of liver damage was evaluated by determination of serum enzyme activities (GOT, GPT, SDH) 24 hours (praseodymium 72 hours) after intraperitoneal injection of the hepatotoxic agents. Body weight of the mice declined by 23% and liver weight by 29% after 24 hours food deprivation. Fasting strongly enhanced the hepatotoxic effects of carbon tetrachloride (0.02 ml/kg), paracetamol (350 mg/kg), thioacetamide (35 mg/kg), and bromobenzene (0.25 ml/kg). The hepatotoxic actions of phalloidine (1.5 mg/kg) and allyl alcohol (0.1 ml/kg) were only increased moderately, and those of α-amanitine (0.75 mg/kg) and praseodymium (200 mg/kg) not at all. In rats, 24-hours fasting enhanced the hepatotoxic action of carbon tetrachloride (0.1 ml/kg), too. Feeding a protein-free diet during 24 hours, however, did not enhance carbon tetrachloride-induced hepatotoxicity in mice. 24-hours fasting increased p-hydroxylation of aniline in the 9000 · g supernatant of mouse liver homogenate from 2.24 ± 0.13 to 3.31 ± 0.18 μmol/g liver and diminished glutathione concentration in the mouse liver from 4.26 ± 0.35 to 1.96 ± 0.52 μmol/g liver. The enhanced hepatotoxic response after fasting is presumably due to 1) a higher conversion rate of the hepatotoxines to toxic metabolites and 2) a lower detoxification rate (conjugation with glutathione).

Abteilung für Toxikologie, Medizinische Hochschule, Ratzeburger Allee 160, D-2400 Lübeck

73

ON THE DEVELOPMENT OF TOLERANCE TO HEPATOTOXIC AGENTS O. Strubelt and M. Völpel

The strong increment of serum enzyme levels (GOT, GPT, SDH) occurring in rats 24 hours after oral administration of 1 g/kg paracetamol vanished completely when the same dose was given once daily for 4 days. This tolerance to paracetamol-induced hepatotoxicity was confirmed by histopathological as well as functional (bromsulphthaleine retention) examination of the livers. Treatment with 3 doses of 1 g/kg paracetamol daily diminished also the hepatotoxic effects of carbon tetrachloride, bromobenzene and thioacetamide, respectively. From the determination of paracetamol concentrations (free and conjugated) in plasma, liver and urine it became evident that the development of tolerance was not due to changes in the pharmacokinetics of paracetamol. Furthermore, the antiphlogistic activity of paracetamol (carrageenin rat paw edema) was not attenuated after subacute treatment with the drug. Microsomal aniline hydroxylase activity, however, decreased by about 30% after subacute paracetamol treatment. From this result it can be concluded that paracetamol-induced protection against paracetamol hepatotoxicity is due to a lower conversion rate of the compound to the proposed arylating N-hydroxymetabolite. Tolerance to hepatotoxicity also developed within 3 to 4 days during daily oral treatment with 0.25 ml/kg bromobenzene, 50 mg/kg thioacetamide or 0.07 ml/kg allyl alcohol, respectively, and was also reported to occur after repeated dosage of carbon tetrachloride (A.E. Glende, Biochem. Pharmacol. 21, 1697; 1972).

Abteilung für Toxikologie, Medizinische Hochschule, Ratzeburger Allee 160, D-2400 Lübeck

74

LIVER DAMAGE BY COUMARIN? W. Drommer[1], W. Endell[3], E.D. Kreuser[2] and G. Seidel[3]

As coumarin is used as flavouring agent for human food as well in the treatment of angiological diseases toxic and - in rats - even cancerogenic effects of the drug should be considered carefully. However, since in rats its metabolism results mainly in hydroxyphenylcarbonic acids but in man mainly in 7-hydroxycoumarin, the rat seems to be unsuitable for studies related to coumarin side effects in man. Therefore the toxicity of coumarin was studied in DBA/2J-mice, having high coumarin-hydroxylase activity in the liver as man, and CH3/HeJ-mice, having low activity as rats. The LD50 of orally administered olive oil dissolved coumarin was found to be double as high in male DBA- than in male CH3-mice (780 and 420 mg/kg; parallel dose effect curves). The oral administration of 350 mg/kg coumarin increased the serum GOT and SDH in CH3-mice to higher levels than in the other strain. Up to 32 weeks feeding with 0.5 and even 1.0% of coumarin in standard diet was tolerated without any impairment of the mice's attitude and growth. 10, 20 and 32 weeks administration of 0.5% coumarin in the diet did not have any effect on the serum levels of GOT, γ-GT and SDH. 1.0% of coumarin, i.e. up to 2 g/kg·day, caused only minimal and irregular increases of one or two enzymes. However, light and - as far as done - electron microscopy did not reveal any consequences in direction to coumarin caused liver damage. - Careful and previous extrapolation of these results to man does not exhibit any important risk of coumarin containing foodstuffs or remedies.

[1]Abtl. Pathol. der Tierärztl. Hochschule Hannover, Abtl. [2]Pathol./[3]Pharmakol. der Med. Hochschule, Ratzeburger Allee 160, D-2400 Lübeck

75

INFLUENCE OF ANTIDOTES ON THE PARACETAMOL-INDUCED THIOETHER EXCRETION IN RATS C.-P. Siegers

The postulated hepatotoxic metabolite of paracetamol is conjugated to cysteine and glutathione. We now studied the influence of 4 antidotes previously found to protect rats and mice against paracetamol-induced liver damage on the renal excretion of thioethers (Ellman's test) and of paracetamol mercapturate (high-pressure liquid chromatography). Urinary thioether excretion in rats ($\bar{x} \pm s_{\bar{x}}$; n = 6 each) was as follows:

Treatment	Dose g/kg	μmol SH/mmol creatinine alone	+ 1g/kg Paracetamol p.o.
Controls	-	230 + 30	
Paracetamol p.o.	1.0	530 + 130	-
DMSO i.p.	1.0	220 + 20	420 + 110
Cysteine i.p.	0.2	300 + 40	800 + 220
Cysteamine i.p.	0.1	1040 + 30	1340 + 220
Dithiocarb i.p.	0.1	5100 + 990	5820 + 1230

Cysteine and DMSO had no significant influence on paracetamol-induced thioether excretion; the strong own effects of cysteamine and dithiocarb masked their action. The excretion of the mercapturic acid conjugate of paracetamol was reduced from 2.41% to 0.8% of dose by treatment with dithiocarb; the 3 other antidotes did not influence the excretion of paracetamol-mercapturate. These results agree with our hypothesis that dithiocarb inhibits the activation of paracetamol by depressing mixed-function oxidase activity.

Abteilung für Toxikologie, Medizinische Hochschule, Ratzeburger Allee 160, D-2400 Lübeck

76

RESPONSE OF PHOSPHOLIPID METABOLISM TO THIRAM IN RAT LIVER MICROSOMES
S. Leyck and K.J. Freundt

Thiurams are potential inhibitors of hepatic mixed-function oxidases (MFO) in experimental animals and man. The underlying mechanism is largely unknown. The present investigations were designed to elucidate this inhibitory effect. Adult female Wistar rats received thiram (tetramethylthiuramdisulfide, a fungicide and rubber accelerator), 1 g/kg by stomach tube, as a suspension in gum arabic and sucrose. After 16 h the livers were subjected to extracorporeal perfusion for 1 h, the perfusate containing ca. 10 μCi u ^{14}C glucose/100 ml. Incorporation of ^{14}C into the phospholipid components of the liver microsomes isolated by a conventional method was determined quantitatively using β-scintillation measurement after preceding TLC separation. The percentage incorporation of ^{14}C into respectively lysophosphatidylcholine, sphingomyelins, and phosphatidylinositol was enhanced, phosphatidylserine remaining uninfluenced. ^{14}C incorporation into phosphatidylcholine and phosphatidylethanolamine was most strikingly depressed by about 1/3. This effect correlated strongly with an inhibition of MFO as shown by a decrease in the O-demethylation of p-nitroanisol in prepared liver microsomes. It is concluded that the reduced turnover of phosphatidylcholine, which is essential to membrane-bound electron transport, contributes to the inhibitory effect on the molecular level. (Supported by a grant from the DFG)

Institute of Pharmacology and Toxicology, Faculty of Clinical Medicine Mannheim, University of Heidelberg, Maybachstrasse 14-16, D-6800 Mannheim.

77

INFLUENCE OF PARAQUAT ON MICROSOMAL OXYGEN UPTAKE   Ch. Steffen

Lipid peroxidation by activated forms of oxygen has been proposed as a mechanism of paraquat (PQ) toxicity by Bus et al. (Environm. Hlth.Perspect. 16, 139, 1976). These authors demonstrated increased peroxidation of microsomal lipids by PQ as measured by formation of malondialdehyde (MDA), whereas other authors found inhibition (Montgomery, Tox.appl.Pharmacol. 36, 543, 1976; Jlett et al., ibid. 28, 216, 1974). In mice liver microsomes the NADPH dependent oxygen uptake is increased by PQ in a dose dependent manner. The observed K_m of 3.10^{-4} M for PQ shows a relatively low affinity of PQ to the sensitive site. In contrast, MDA formation is inhibited with a lower concentration of PQ (K_i: 6.10^{-5} M) Other inhibitors of MDA formation such as EDTA, catechol, neotetrazolium do not influence the PQ-induced oxygen consumption. Induction by phenobarbitone increases the PQ-induced oxygen consumption but not the formation of MDA, suggesting a role for NADPH-cytochrome c-reductase as does also the insensitivity to CO. In the presence of PQ 2 moles of NADPH were oxidized per mole oxygen, while in its absence the ratio was close to 1. Oxidation of methanol to formaldehyde was enhanced by PQ. The above PQ effects are similar to those of menadione, which is a substrate of NADPH-cytochrome c-reductase (Nishibayashi et al., Biochem.Biophys.Acta 67, 520, 1963) and is effective in much lower concentrations with a NADPH/oxygen ratio of 1. These results are consistent with an increased formation of hydrogen peroxide by PQ and the subsequent cleavage to oxygen and water by catalase. Under our experimental conditions a divergence between MDA formation and oxygen consumption - both are considered as parameters of lipid peroxidation - becomes obvious.

This work was supported by the Deutsche Forschungsgemeinschaft, Bonn - Bad Godesberg.

Department of Pharmacology and Toxicology, University of Marburg, Lahnberge, D-3550 Marburg

78

PEROXIDATION OF MITOCHONDRIAL LIPIDS OF RAT LIVER FOLLOWING CHRONIC AND ACUTE ALCOHOL TREATMENT
J. Haselbach, E. Pfaff, and H. Remmer

Liver mitochondria were isolated from normal or alcohol treated rats. Their susceptibility to lipid peroxidation (LPO) on Fe-ADP addition was studied by following malondialdehyde production. Chronic alcohol dosing (3 weeks) resulted in a decreased LPO (initial rates less than half). In vitro additions of ethanol to normal mitochondria enhanced LPO, almost doubling initial rates at 2 ^{o}/oo, whereas mitochondria from chronically treated animals showed little effect. Furthermore, chronic treatment decreased mitochondrial coupling as measured by the acceptor control ratio (ACR). In vitro additions had no effect. On alcohol treatment, the decreases in LPO and ACR showed individual, but parallel variations; for a given substrate, a close correlation of both parameters could be shown. Since the ACR reflects the maximum capability of a mitochondrial preparation for membrane energization brought about by charge separation due to respiration, we studied the effects of respiratory inhibitors and effectors of the surface charge density of the membrane. Respiratory inhibition by antimycin A or KCN almost halved LPO. Atractyloside or bromosulfophthalein which increased the negative surface charge by binding to the mitochondrial membrane enhanced LPO. LPO in mitochondria from chronically treated animals - though at lower levels - was affected analogously. The dependence of LPO on the energizeability of the mitochondrial membrane can also be demonstrated by titration with an uncoupler resulting in a decrease in ACR by successive increases in the proton permeability of the membrane and,consequently, decreased energizeability. Again, decreases in ACR and LPO were correlated.

Department of Toxicology, University of Tübingen, Wilhelmstrasse 56, D-7400 Tübingen

79

INFLUENCE OF DIET AND XENOBIOTICS ON THE URINARY EXCRETION OF BOUND THIOL GROUPS IN MAN AND RATS   R. Pentz

The urinary excretion of bound thiol groups, measured with the method of G.L. Ellman (Arch. Biochem. 82, 70; 1959) was claimed recently to be a parameter for the exposition to alkylating agents (F. Seutter-Berlage et al., Int. Arch. Occup. Environm. Hlth 39, 45; 1977). In 103 ambulant patients of our hospital excretion of bound SH-groups ranged between 7 and 314 (mean value 68) µmol/mmol creatinine. In patients with high values no apparent relation to medication or the state of health was found. A long-time study in four healthy volunteers revealed intraindividual changes of thioether-excretion by at least 100%. One person excreted very high amounts of thioether (100 to 175 µmol SH/mmol creatinine) without any evidence for a high exposition to alkylating agents.
The 24-h-urine of male wistar rats contained 13.5 ±1.3 µmol bound SH groups = 200 ±11 µmol SH/mmol creatinine. At least 50% of this basic value was excreted even by rats which had been starved for 3 days or fed glucose as sole food for 4 days. This indicates a relatively high excretion of endogenous substrates as thioethers. Treatment of rats with toxic doses of 35 compounds including 17 carcinogens caused an increase of thioether excretion in only 13 cases. Strong carcinogens and alkylating substances, e.g. N-nitrosoamines, dimethylsulfate and benzopyrene, had no significant influence. Our investigation doubts the value of Ellman's test as an indicator for the exposition to xenobiotics.

Abteilung für Toxikologie, Medizinische Hochschule, Ratzeburger Allee 160, D-2400 Lübeck

80

DIFFERENCES IN BINDING OF NITROSAMINES TO CYTOCHROM P 450. POSSIBLE RELEVANCE FOR THEIR ACTIVATION AND INACTIVATION. K.E.Appel and H.W.Kunz.

Previous investigations showed a decrease in alkylation rate and a reduced carcinogenic efficiency of diethyl- and dimethylnitrosamine (DMN) due to induction of microsomal monoxigenase system. These findings are incomprehensible with the commonly accepted activation mechanism of nitrosamines if their oxidative desalkylation is increased after induction as it is normally known for other Cyt.P450 dependent reactions. This was confirmed for DMN by several investigators. Using low DMN doses,however, a depression of DMN-demythylase activity following phenobarbital- and 3-MC-induction was reported. In agreement with these results we found that inhibition or increase of demethylation and the corresponding alkylation are dependent on DMN concentration. Studying the causes of this phenomenon we obtained evidence, that nitrosamines can bind as substrates as well as ligands to Cyt.P 450. Phenobarbital induced mice liver microsomes showed typical type I spectral characteristics with DMN and other dialkylnitrosamines in concentrations of 1-5 mM. With diphenylnitrosamine(DPhNA), however, a ligand spectrum with a maximum about 439 nm was obtained. Microsomes from 3-MC-treated rats produced ligand spectra only with all nitrosamines tested showing maxima between 42o and 440 nm. After reduction with dithionite the resulting difference spectra showed peaks with varying extents between 445 and 455 nm. CO and metyrapone seem to be unable to displace the exogenous ligand of the nitrosamin P 450 complex. Therefore, recording the reduced CO difference spectra one can obtain an evaluation of the amount of Cyt.P 450 able to complex with nitrosamine. We found that the extent of the reduced ligand complex formation depends on nitrosamine derivate, sex and species of animals and type of P 450 inducer; e.g.80% resp.15% of P 450 shows a ligand binding with DPhNA resp. DMN. If this ligand binding is of any relevance for the observed reduced metabolic activation of nitrosamines after induction will be further investigated.

German Cancer Research Center, Dpt. molec. Toxicology, D-6900 Heidelberg

81

METABOLISM AND SUBCELLULAR EFFECTS OF DIMETHYLNITRO-
SAMINE INCUBATED IN VITRO WITH ISOLATED LIVER CELLS

Michael Schwarz and Renate Rickart

Rat liver parenchymal cells were isolated enzymatically
and incubated in vitro in suspension or monolayer. In
the course of incubation time synthesis rate of DNA
and different RNA-species as well as cytochrome contents and function of microsomal monooxygenase system
were determined.

To study the metabolic activation of ^{14}C-Dimethylnitro-
samine (DMN) CH_2O-formation, specific activities of
cellular macromolecules and base alkylation of RNA and
DNA were measured.

As a suitable parameter of carcinogen-induced DNA
alterations the amount of single strand breaks following in vivo application or in vitro incubation of
DMN and N-Methyl-N'-nitro-N-nitrosoguanidine (MNNG)
were determined. The methods used for quantification
of DNA-strand breaks, e.g. velocity sedimentation in
alkaline sucrose gradients, and alkaline filter elu-
tion will be demonstrated.

German Cancer Research Center, Dept. of Molecular
Toxicology, Im Neuenheimer Feld 280, D-6900 Heidelberg

82

LOSS OF TWO-STAGE-CONTROL OF CELL PROLIFERATION IN
RAT LIVER AFTER A SINGLE DOSE OF THE CARCINOGEN
DIETHYLNITROSAMINE R. Schulte Hermann

Stimulation of liver cell proliferation in adoles-
cent rats by endogenous stimuli or by xenobiotic
compounds such as phenobarbital, α-hexachlorocyclo-
hexane (α-HCH) etc. is controlled by a Two-Stage
mechanism: After initiation of the replicative process by the growth stimulus (first signal) a second
signal is required which is provided by consumption
of protein-containing food. In the absence of
dietary protein cells programmed for replication are
arrested some hours before commencement of DNA synthesis [R. Schulte Hermann, Cancer Res. 37, 166
(1977)].
This mechanism is disturbed after administration of
diethylnitrosamine (DENA): proliferating cells are
no longer arrested by protein deprivation but escape
from this restriction. These observations may prove
useful for the early detection of preneoplastic
lesions. In addition they may provide a tool for
further studies on the promotion of liver tumor
formation by inducers of liver growth such as phenobarbital, HCH, DDT etc.

Institut für Toxikologie und Pharmakologie,
Philipps Universität Marburg/Lahn, D 355 Marburg,
Pilgrimstein 2

83

ALKYLATING AND MUTAGENIC EFFECTS OF ALLYL AND
ALLYLOGENIC COMPOUNDS   E.Eder and T.Neudecker

Some allyl compounds have been found active,
others inactive in carcinogenicity testing in
intact animals. The carcinogenic activity has
been attributed, up to now, to the possible
epoxidation of the olefinic moiety in these
molecules. However, allylic or allylogenic structures are generally characterized by a rather
strong S_N-1 as well as S_N-2 reactivity; they may
alkylate nucleophilic biomolecules and thus
initiate chemical carcinogenesis and mutagenesis.
We investigated the direct alkylating properties
of a series of allyl and allylogenic compounds
and tested their mutagenic potential in an in
vitro-bacterial testing system (A) (Ames et al.,
Proc.Natl.Sci.70,2281;1973). - The selection of
compounds was guided by theoretical evaluation
of the influence of various substituents on the
reactivity of the molecules. These alkylating
properties were determined by reaction with 4-
nitrobenzyl pyridine (B). Positive results in A
and B were found with: allyl chloride, allyl
cyanide, 1-chloro-2-methyl-2-propene, 1-chloro-
2-butene; negative, in both tests (A and B) were
allyl amine and diallyl sulfide. With allyl alcohol, a high mutagenic potential (A) did not
correlate with a negative result in B; this, however, might be due to the fact that OH, under
the condition of test, does not represent a good
leaving group. These findings clearly indicate
the possibility that allyl compounds might exert
a direct carcinogenic effect. Whether or not
this competes with an epoxidation as an indirect
activating mechanism is due to further investigations.

Department of Toxicology, University of Würzburg,
D-8700 Würzburg, Versbacher Landstraße 9

84

ALKYLATION OF DNA AND RNA BY METABOLITES OF
VINYL CHLORIDE AND VINYL BROMIDE.
R.J.Laib and H.Ottenwälder

If rats are exposed to ^{14}C-vinyl chloride, radioactivity is incorporated into nucleic acids of
the liver. In previous investigations (Toxicology
8,185,1977) we showed incorporation of radioactivity from ^{14}C-vinyl chloride into the physiological bases of RNA. In addition, alkylation of
adenosine and cytidine moieties occurred leading
to formation of radioactive 1,N^6-ethenoadenosine
and 3,N^4-ethenocytidine. The time courses of
1,N^6-ethenoadenosine and 3,N^4-ethenocytidine in
rat liver RNA after vinyl chloride inhalation
are dissimilar: 92 hrs after ending exposure the
ethenoadenosine is only 1/5 of its original value
whereas the content of ethenocytidine persists.
This ought to be indicative for the relative
importance of cytidine alkylation. Formation of
labelled etheno derivatives of adenosine and cytidine was also observed if rats were exposed to
[14]C-vinyl bromide. To establish possible changes
in DNA due to alkylation by vinyl chloride metabolites, DNA was incubated with rat liver microsomes, NADPH and ^{14}C-vinyl chloride. Re-isolation
of the DNA, hydrolysis and separation of the nucleosides on Aminex-A-6 showed that small amounts
of radioactive 1,N^6-etheno 2'deoxyadenosine and
3,N^4-etheno 2'deoxycytidine were formed. Besides,
a major alkylation product, presumably of 2'deoxy
guanosine was isolated which, on Aminex-A-6-
columns, showed the same chromatographic behavior
as a compound which was obtained from chemical
reaction of 2'deoxyguanosine with chloroacetalde-
hyde.

Institut für Toxikologie, Universität Tübingen,
Wilhelmstraße 56, D-7400 Tübingen

85
PHARMACOKINETICS OF HALOGENATED ETHYLENES

J.G.Filser and H.M.Bolt

The present discussion of toxic effects of vinyl chloride raises the question of interpretation of toxicological data. Evidently, biochemical and mechanistic concepts of action of halogenated ethylenes can only be correlated with toxicities observed in vivo, if differences in pharmacokinetics are taken into account. This consideration led to the present investigation. Rats were exposed in a closed system to atmospheric concentrations of fluoroethylene (vinyl fluoride) 1,1-difluoroethylene (vinylidene fluoride), chloroethylene (vinyl chloride), 1,1-dichloroethylene (vinylidene chloride), trans- and cis-1,2-dichloroethylene, trichloroethylene, and bromoethylene (vinyl bromide). Pharmacokinetic analysis was done as previously described (Toxicology $\underline{7}$, 179, 1977). The following principles could be derived. (1)"Non-linear"(dose-dependent) pharmacokinetics may apply if the organism is exposed to higher concentrations of halogenated ethylenes. This is constsient with the concept of Watanabe, Young & Gehring (J.Env.Path.Tox.$\underline{1}$, 1977). In the case of vinyl chloride, it refers to atmospheric concentrations higher than 250 ppm. (2) The equilibrium constant of distribution of the non-metabolised compound (concentration in the animal/concentration in the gas phase) increases from vinyl fluoride to vinyl bromide. (3) The rate of metabolism depends on the structural properties of the individual compound. Trans-1,2-dichloroethylene and vinylidene fluoride are extremely slowly metabolised, comparable to the rate of metabolism of 1,1,1-trichloroethane (methyl chloroform) which was used as a reference compound.

Institut für Toxikologie, Universität Tübingen.

86
METABOLISM OF HALOTHANE AS A FUNCTION OF SUBSTRATE CONCENTRATION IN THE ISOLATED PERFUSED RAT LIVER PREPARATION

I. Rösch and E. Dallmeier

Halothane (H) is metabolically converted mainly to trifluoroacetic acid (TFA). Whilst in surgical anaesthesia the proportion metabolised has been determined at 15-20%, we found in long-term exposure of volunteers to environmental concentrations (8-50 ppm) a proportion of 60-70% (Dallmeier and Henschler,Arch.Pharmac.$\underline{297}$,R 20; 1977). To elucidate the reason for this gap we initiated experiments with the isolated perfused rat liver by offering steady-state concentrations ranging from 13 to 3200 ppm (gas phase) via the oxygenator. The difference of H-concentrations before and after liver passage was taken as amount metabolised, liver function was checked by standard enzyme tests. Metabolization rate (in terms of nMole $H \cdot g^{-1}$ liver$\cdot min^{-1}$) increases from 0.36 (13 ppm H) to 16.5 (3200 ppm), corresponding to proportions of conversion of 97% and 15%,respectively. Lineweaver-Burk plot reveals a linear relationship between reciprocals of metabolization rate and H-concentration, half saturation of the rate limiting step being calculated at 600 ppm H (gas phase). The ratio of TFA formed to the amount H metabolised is close to unity at low concentration ranges, with a distinct tendency to decrease towards higher H concentrations. It is concluded that biomonitoring of TFA-levels in blood or urine can be taken representative of H load only in the range of very low H-concentrations.

Department of Toxicology, University of Würzburg, Versbacher Landstraße 9, D-8700 Würzburg

87
DISPOSITION AND METABOLISM OF $[^{14}C]$ 1,1-DICHLOROETHYLENE AFTER SINGLE ORAL ADMINISTRATION IN RATS

D. Reichert and H.W. Werner

1,1-Dichloroethylene (VDC, vinylidene chloride) is converted metabolically to mutagenic and carcinogenic intermediates. We have investigated the metabolic fate of ^{14}C-VDC in rats after single oral doses of 0.5; 5 and 50 mg/kg by collecting and analysing expired air, urine and feces for 72 hours following administration. The proportions of expired unchanged VDC/$^{14}CO_2$/ urinary activity were as follows: 0.5 mg/kg-0.9%/23%/52%; 50 mg/kg-20%/6%/36%. This change in the conversion rate and in the pattern of metabolites is indicative of a rapid saturation of VDC metabolism. This is consistent with previous studies on the uptake and metabolism of VDC by the isolated perfused rat liver (Reichert et al., Int.Arch.Occ.Envir.Hlth 1978, in press).
Non-volatile radioactivity within the body after 72 hr comprised 2-4% of the administered dose and was highest in the liver, the other organs containing minimal amounts only. Thus, most of the VDC is rapidly excreted either unchanged or in the form of polar metabolites. Three major metabolites were separated by thin layer chromatography and gas chromatography, the main part of activity has been identified as thiodiglycolic acid by mass spectrometry.

Department of Toxicology, University of Würzburg, Versbacher Landstraße 9, D-8700 Würzburg

88
ON THE METABOLIC FORMATION OF CARBON MONOXIDE FROM TRICHLOROETHYLENE

H. Fetz, W.R. Hoos and D. Henschler

Dichloromethane (CH_2Cl_2) is metabolically converted to carbon monoxide (CO) (Kubic et al., Drug Metabol.Disp.$\underline{2}$,53;1974). Traylor et al. (Hoppe-Seyler's Z.$\overline{357}$,1060;1976) postulated a similar reaction with trichloroethylene (Tri) by using an in vitro microsomal system; they determined CO indirectly as carboxyhemoglobin. Doubts arose since in intact animals no CO is formed under Tri inhalation (unpublished), and in previous experiments with rabbit liver microsomes a typical P-450 binding spectrum was found which is similar to but distinctly different from that with CO (Uehleke et al.,Arch.Toxicol.$\underline{37}$,95; 1977). - We reinvestigated this problem by introducing a GC microdetermination of CO. The typical P-450 binding spectrum was reproduced with Tri and microsomes from livers of mice, rats and rabbits (λ_{max}=451-2 nm). Traces of CO were detectable in all experiments, also in controls without addition of Tri; this background formation of CO is most probably due to heme degradation (Wolff & Bidlack,Biochem.Biophys.Res.Comm.$\underline{73}$,850;1976). - Pure Tri-oxirane produced a typical CO spectrum with microsomes (λ_{max}=450 nm), and large amounts of CO have been found. It is suggested that Tri-oxirane may, under certain conditions, decompose in part to CO; under in vivo conditions of Tri-oxidation, however, the intermediate oxirane is rapidly and completely rearranged to chloral hydrate (Bonse & Henschler, Crit.Rev.Toxicol.$\underline{4}$,395;1976) without CO formation.

Department of Toxicology, University of Würzburg, Versbacher Landstraße 9, D-8700 Würzburg

89

EFFECT OF ANTIOXIDANTS ON IRREVERSIBLE BINDING OF CCl_4 TO PROTEINS AND LIPIDS IN RAT LIVER MICROSOMES COMPARED TO LIPID PEROXIDATION, H. Kieczka

In microsomal systems CCl_4 is activated to a radical by which lipids from rat liver microsomes are peroxidated. The formation of lipid peroxides is accompanied by the irreversible binding of CCl_4 to microsomal proteins and lipids which is highest under anaerobic conditions.
When liposomes from egg lecithine were incubated with cytochrome c reductase, a NADPH-regenerating system and CCl_4, no formation of malondialdehyde (MDA) was observed. This result allows the conclusion that cytochrome c reductase is not involved in the activation step of CCl_4. Furthermore, we incubated rat liver microsomes (2 mg protein/ml) with a NADPH-regenerating system and CCl_4 under different pO_2 and determined simultaneously the formation of MDA and the irreversible binding of CCl_4 to lipids and proteins. At low concentrations of O_2 we measured a higher MDA formation than by higher pO_2. The optimal O_2 concentration which was used in the present experiments was found to be 5 % in the gaseous phase.
We found that lipid peroxidation as well as irreversible binding of CCl_4 to proteins and lipids were inhibited by antioxidants with catechol structure. In all cases a 50 % inhibition (I_{50}) was observed in concentrations of the same order of magnitude: Propylgallate, $I_{50} = 6 \times 10^{-6}$ M; 2-hydroxy-Estradiol, $I_{50} = 4 \times 10^{-6}$ M. We found that the relationship of irreversible binding of CCl_4 to proteins and lipids is changed by increasing concentrations of catechol antioxidants (1×10^{-6} to 5×10^{-5} M). This relationship shifts from 1 : 3 to 1 : 0.7.

Institut für Toxikologie der Universität Tübingen, Wilhelmstraße 56, D 7400 Tübingen

90

APPLICATION OF A BIOASSAY FOR THE DETERMINATION OF PICOGRAM LEVELS OF 2,3,7,8-TETRACHLORODIBENZO-p-DIOXIN (TCDD). F.J. Wiebel and I. Gebefügi

TCDD is a powerful inducer of aryl hydrocarbon (benzo(a)pyrene) hydroxylase (AHH) in vivo and in vitro (Poland and Glover, Mol. Pharmacol. 10,349, 1974; Niwa et al.,Mol. Pharmacol. 11,399,1975). In the rat hepatoma cell line, H-4-II-E, TCDD elicits half-maximum AHH induction at a concentration of about 15 pg/ml growth medium.

AHH induction was utilized to study the photodegradation of TCDD under simulated environmental conditions. Under exposure to light filtered by Quartz ($\lambda > 230$nm) or "Pyrex"-glass ($\lambda > 290$nm) TCDD is degraded with a half life of 1/2 and 1 day,respectively. These results were in agreement with parallel gaschromatographic determinations. The findings suggest that the photodegradation products do not interfere with the induction bioassay of the parent compound.

TCDD could also be measured using the induction assay when adsorbed to silica gel (70-230 mesh) or to soil. Thus, addition of not more than 10 mg of wet soil containing 2 μg TCDD/kg to 1 ml of growth medium caused about half-maximum induction of AHH. Based on these findings we have begun to test soil samples from the Seveso area. A few mg of unprocessed soil obtained from the heavily contaminated area (zone A) strongly induced AHH whereas soil samples from the surrounding area (zone B) showed no significant effect. Our results indicate that the induction of AHH in culture may provide a facile and highly sensitive tool to probe for the presence of TCDD in the environment.

Abtl. Toxikologie and Inst. Oekolog.Chemie, Gesellschaft für Strahlen u. Umweltforschung, D-8042 Neuherberg/München

91

STUDIES ON THE MECHANISM OF IRREVERSIBLE PROTEIN-BINDING OF AROMATIC HYDROCARBONS, MEDIATED BY RAT LIVER MICROSOMES: BINDING OF ^{14}C-NAPHTHALENE AND ^{14}C-1-NAPHTHOL. S.Hesse and M.Mezger

Previous results suggested that the irreversible protein binding of polychlorinated biphenyls (PCBs) in the presence of rat liver microsomes is caused not only by the primary oxidation products, epoxides, but also by some secondary reactive metabolite(s) (S.Hesse et al.,Chem.Biol.Interact.in press). In this study we wanted to examine, whether this might apply to the binding of other aromatic hydrocarbons. ^{14}C-Naphthalene and ^{14}C-1-naphthol, a major product of microsomal metabolism, served as "model" substrates.Both compounds were irreversible bound to microsomal protein, when incubated with rat liver microsomes and a NADPH-generating system. The binding rate of ^{14}C-naphthalene was stimulated to a minor extent by pretreatment of the rats with phenobarbital (PB) or 3-methylcholanthrene (3-MC). In vitro addition of 0.2-0.4 mM trichloropropene oxide (TCPO) only slightly increased the binding of ^{14}C-naphthalene. The binding was inhibited by 85% in the presence of 0.5 mM SKF 525 A and also in the presence of 3 mM UDP-glucuronic acid, which reduces the concentration of free naphthol. In contrast the binding of ^{14}C-naphthol was doubled by using microsomes of PB- or 3-MC- treated rats. SKF and TCPO did not affect the binding of ^{14}C-naphthol. The results are compatible with the notion that during secondary metabolism of naphthalene, i.e. oxidation of phenolic metabolites "reactive" intermediates are formed which greatly contribute to the "overall" binding.

Gesellschaft f. Strahlen- und Umweltforschung, Abtlg. Toxikologie, D-8042 Neuherberg/München.

92

EFFECT OF MONOOXYGENASE INDUCERS ON THE BINDING OF BENZO-(A)PYRENE METABOLITES TO CELLULAR MACROMOLECULES IN PERFUSED RAT LUNGS E. Klaus, B. Deckers-Schmelzle, and G.F. Kahl

The irreversible binding of metabolically activated [^{3}H]-benzo(a)pyrene (BP) to cellular macromolecules of isolated perfused rat lungs was studied. Lungs from differently pretreated animals were perfused in situ in a recirculating system without ventilation. BP with a specific activity of 10 mCi/μmol was added to 50 ml perfusion medium containing 40% washed bovine erythrocytes to a final concentration of 1 μM. DNA, RNA and protein fractions were isolated and assayed for irreversibly bound radioactivity.

Pretreatment of the animals with the inducer of cytochrome P-448, ß-naphthoflavone, increased irreversible binding to cellular constituents by a factor of 15 to 25. In lungs of induced animals, 0.5 pmoles BP equivalents were bound per mg of DNA, 2.5 pmoles per mg of RNA and 7.6 pmoles BP equivalents per mg of protein. A slight increase in binding was also found after pretreatment with the cytochrome P-450 inducer phenobarbital but was statistically not significant. This is different to what was found in liver perfusion experiments (G.F. Kahl et al., Arch. Toxicol., in press) since in the liver binding to DNA could also be increased by phenobarbital pretreatment.

Department of Pharmacology, University of Mainz, Obere Zahlbacher Str. 67, D-6500 Mainz

93

ADENYLATE CYCLASE FROM GUINEA-PIG BRAIN:
STUDIES OF A NUCLEOTIDE BINDING PROTEIN
A. du Moulin, J. Schultz

Guanylylimidodiphosphate (GMP-PNP) influences the
adenylate cyclase activity in almost all tissues.
There are investigations of GMP-PNP binding to
avian erythrocyte membranes (A.M. Spiegel, G.D.
Aurbach J.Biol.Chem. 249 7630 (1974), T. Pfeuffer
E. Helmreich J.Biol.Chem. 250 867 (1975)) trying
to relate GMP-PNP binding to the activation of
adenylate cyclase. Since ATP is normally abundant
within a cell and is the substrate of adenylate
cyclase, we investigated the binding of ^{3}H-ATP to
a particulate and Lubrol-PX solubilized membrane
preparation. Both of these possess adenylate cyclase activity. A Scatchard plot reveals a high
($K=2,0 \times 10^7$/M) and a low ($K=2,6 \times 10^6$/M) affinity constant, very similar in both preparations.
These binding sites are, however, not the substrate binding sites which have an association
constant of 6×10^5/M. Treatment of the particulate membrane fraction with hypotonic buffer re-
leases an ATP binding protein (heat labile, sensitive to freezing) that has two binding sites
with the above association constants. It could be
separated from phosphodiesterase activity and the
known calcium dependent regulator by chromatographic procedures. GMP-PNP influences the ATP binding to the particulate and the solubilized preparations. Because GMP-PNP also has two binding
sites (A.M. Spiegel) -of which only the low affinity site differs from the ATP binding data- we
speculate that our protein may be related to the
GMP-PNP binding protein as mentioned above and
may be involved in the regulation of adenylate
cyclase activity of brain.

Pharmazeutisches Institut, Universität Tübingen,
Auf der Morgenstelle.

94

PROSTAGLANDIN-INDUCED cAMP SYNTHESIS IN
PERIPHERAL NERVE   Peter Kalix

Prostaglandins of the E series induce an acceleration
of cAMP synthesis in peripheral nerve tissue from several species. For example, exposure to PE 1 increases
the cAMP content in calf vagus nerve twofold and in
that of the rabbit threefold; PE 2 has a comparable
effect. Similarly, PE 1 increases the cAMP synthesis
in the superior cervical ganglion of calf, rat and
rabbit; in these tissues, however, the presence of a
phosphodiesterase inhibitor is required for accumulation of the nucleotide.

Rabbit vagus nerves were used to investigate some of
the characteristics of the observed effect. The action
of PE 1 is rapid (1-5 min), it can be elicited by 1 µM
and is maximal at 10 µM PE 1. Prostaglandins of the A,
B and F series do not induce cAMP synthesis in a manner
comparable to that of PE 1 or PE 2. Polyphloretin phosphate and 7-oxa-13-prostynoic acid, substances that
interfere with certain responses to prostaglandins, do
not inhibit the stimulation of cAMP synthesis by PE 1.

Département de Pharmacologie de l'Université
CH 1211 Genève 4 (Schweiz)

95

THE EFFECT OF CA AND MG IONS ON THE FORMATION OF
cAMP IN ISOPRENALINE-STIMULATED RESEALED RAT RE-
TICULOCYTE GHOSTS. H. Porzig and M. Schneider

The adrenergic β-receptor - adenylate cyclase system in the membranes of resealed rat reticulocyte ghosts resembles more closely the system observed in intact cells than the one found in membrane fragments: In ghosts prepared by reversal
of hemolysis, in the presence of less than 0,01µM
Ca, the adenylate cyclase is half maximally stimulated by 0,1 µM isoprenaline (Ipr). Ipr concentrations above 10 µM are inhibitory. cAMP formation with 10 µM Ipr is at least 5 times higher
than with 10 mM NaF. Intracellular Gpp(NH)p
(10µM) has only a slight stimulatory effect on
the Ipr-mediated cAMP formation. If the ghosts
are prepared at increasing Ca ion concentrations
(0.08 - 5 µM) the K_M value for Ipr is not affected but its maximal stimulatory effect (efficacy)
on cAMP formation is biphasic. The efficacy decreases as Ca is increased from 0.01 to 0.2 µM.
It is enhanced to values above the control level
as Ca is raised further to 5 µM. The Ca dependency is less pronounced in the presence of intracellular Gpp(NH)p. The minimum in Ipr efficacy
is shifted from ~ 0.1 to ~ 0.7 µM Ca if the Mg ion
concentration at which the ghosts are prepared
is increased from 0.3 to 8 mM. The efficacy of
extracellular NaF in stimulating cAMP accumulation shows a similar biphasic Ca dependency as
it is observed with Ipr. The results suggest
that either the coupling between β-receptor and
adenylate cyclase or the intrinsic activity of
this enzyme or both are Ca-dependent functions
of the ghost cell membrane.

Pharmakologisches Institut, Univ. Bern, CH 3010
Bern, Friedbühlstr. 49

96

DISSOCIATION BETWEEN ACTIVITY OF ADENYLCYCLASE
AND DENSITY OF ADRENERGIC β-RECEPTORS DURING
MATURATION OF RAT ERYTHROCYTES
G. Kaiser, J. Dietz, M. Hellwich

β-Adrenergic receptor sites as well as adenylcyclase activity are located preferentially in
immature red blood cells from rats. When the degree of reticulocytosis by treating the animals
with graded doses of acetylphenylhydrazine (3x15
- 70 mg/kg APH) is increased density of adrenergic β-receptors as measured by binding of (-) ^{3}H-
Dihydroalprenolol (DHAP) and adenylcyclase activity are increased in a strong correlation. -
When rats are treated with a constant dose of
APH (3x40 mg/kg) the reticulocyte values increase rapidly from ~2 to ~ 50% reaching a maximum at
the 7th day after the first injection; normal
values are reached again at the 21th day. Basal
and isoprenaline-stimulated synthesis of cAMP in
membrane preparations as well as in intact cells
also increased up to 100 fold during the first
week, beeing normal again at the 21th day after
the first injection. Receptor density increased
up to 4 fold during seven days; thereafter, in
contrast to the rapidly decreasing values of re-
ticulocytes and Vmax-values of isoprenaline stimulated cAMP synthesis β-receptor density decreased rather slowly within two weeks after the
maximum. Dissociation constants for DHAP as well
as the activation constants for isoprenaline as
activator of adenylcyclase remained unchanged. -
    These results indicate that the quantitative
relationship between β-receptors and adenylcyclase changes continuously during the maturation
of the erythrocyte.

Zentrum der Pharmakologie, J.W.Goethe-Universi-
tät, Th.-Stern-Kai 7, D-6000 Frankfurt/Main, FRG

97

SOLUBILIZED CORONARY SMOOTH MUSCLE ADE - NYLYLCYCLASE: INFLUENCE OF LIPIDS ON ADE- NOSINE RESPONSE. I. Rinner, A. Wurm

Previous studies indicated the existence of special adeno- sine (AD) receptors attached to adenylylcyclase(AC) in co- ronary strips (Rinner et al., this journal 297, R 12, 1977). Hence, it was attempted to separate the receptor entity from AC by solubilization of this enzyme, and to recombine both by phospholipid treatment. Solubilization of particu- late AC with either 2 % digitonin or 2 % polyoxyethylene- ether W1 and also prolonged(50 sec) homogenisation of the coronary strips abolished the responsiveness to isoprena- line (IS) and to the stimulant(but not the inhibitory) action of AD, whereas AC remained sensitive to NaF (8 mM)-sti- mulation. Basal activity of the digitonin-solubilized (de- tergent freed) AC was the same as in the particulate pre- paration averaging 4×10^{-10} moles cAMP/mg protein/10 min (measured as ^{32}P-cAMP formed from ^{32}P-ATP in the pre- sence of 1 mM ATP, an ATP regenerating system, cAMP and papaverine). As shown by the percent differences to control activity (tab.), addition of PS to the solubilized AC restored significant(^{x}) stimulant actions of AD (1 nM) and IS (100 nM).

	AD	IS	NaF
Particulate AC	+ 105^x	+ 143^x	+ 261^x
Digitonin-solubilized AC(S)	- 11	- 14	+ 164^x
S + phosphatidylinositol	+ 6	- 5	+ 81^x
S + phosphatidylethanolamine	+ 4	+ 7	+ 136^x
S + phosphatidylserine (PS)	+ 25^x	+ 33^x	+ 131^x

The results indicate the existence of receptors for AD and IS which can be separated from, and reattached to AC.

Inst. f. Pharmakodyn. u. Tox., Univ. Graz, A-8010, Univ. Pl. 2

98

SOLUBLE ADENYLATE CYCLASE AND GUANYLATE CYCLASE IN BOVINE ADRENAL CORTEX: ACTIVATION BY SODIUM NITROPRUSSIDE AND NITROSAMINES - INHIBITION BY PHOSPHOLIPASE A AND FREE FATTY ACIDS C.J.Struck and H. Glossmann

Soluble (100.000xg supernatant) adenylate and guanylate cyclase (sAC, sGC) in bovine adrenal cortex are activated by sodium nitroprusside (SNP) and cancerogens like N-methyl-N-nitro-N-nitroso- guanidin (MNNG). Both enzymatic activities re- side on proteins with similar hydrodynamic pro- perties ($S_{20,w}$-values and Stokes' radii).
A dramatic increase of cGMP levels upon treatment with SNP or MNNG is observed with intact bovine adrenal cells suggesting that activation of sGC by cancerogens and SNP may occur in vivo.
In the presence of unsaturated fatty acids (uFA) and SNP the supernatant looses the ability to convert ATP into cAMP. SNP stimulated sGC is only partially inhibited, in the absence of SNP uFA activate sGC. Saturated FA have no effect. Non- ionic detergents and Lysolecithin interfere with the activation of the cyclases by SNP and MNNG. Phospholipase A (snake venom) treatment of the crude enzyme preparation leads to an abolishment of the SNP activation of sAC.
It is proposed that the cyclases contain a hydro- phobic regulatory site where hydrophobic ligands (e.g. uFA) are bound. We discriminate three func- tional states of the cyclases: A basal state (1) where Mn^{++} is cofactor and GTP is substrate (endo- genous ligands may be bound), a high activity state (2) where Mn^{++} is cofactor for ATP and Mn^{++} or Mg^{++} for GTP, and an intermediate activity state (3) where Mn^{++} is cofactor for GTP. Transitions observed are: (1)→(2) (SNP, MNNG), (1)→(3) (deterg., uFA), (2)→(3) (deterg.,uFA).
Pharmakologisches Institut der JLU Giessen Frankfurter Strasse 107, D-6300 Lahn-Giessen 1

99

Purification And Characterisation Of A cGMP- Dependent Protein Kinase From Bovine Heart Muscle

V. Flockerzi, N. Speichermann, and F. Hofmann

Guanosine 3':5'-momophosphate-dependent protein kinase from bovine heart muscle was purified to apparent homogeneity using affinity chromato- graphy. The kinase activity was purified at least 16.400-fold with an overall recovery of 6%. So- dium dodecyl sulfate gels of purified kinase showed one stained band corresponding to a mole- cular weight of 82.000. When histone I was used as substrate protein, half maximal stimulation of kinase activity by cGMP and cAMP was observed at concentrations of 0.025 and 6.8 M, respective- ly. Low concentrations of magnesium acetate(2mM) were necessary for phosphorylation of histone I. In contrast, optimal phosphorylations rates in the presence of histone IIb (0.2 mg/ml) were ob- tained in the presence of 60 mM magnesium ace- tate. It is suggested, that high concentrations of magnesium are required only for the phosphory- lation of histone IIb.

Pharmakologisches Institut der Universität Hei- delberg, Im Neuenheimer Feld 366, D-6900 Heidel- berg, Germany

100

DECREASED SENSITIVITY OF ß-ADRENOCEPTORS IN LEFT ATRIA FROM HYPOTHYROID RATS. O.-E.Brodde, H.J.Schümann and J.Wagner.

In isolated electrically driven (1.0 Hz, 37°C) left atria of normal rats (NR) as well as of those made hypothyroid (HR) by feeding with propylthiouracil the ß-sympathomimetic effects of isoprenaline (IPN) and of phenylephrine (PE) in the presence of 10^{-5}M yohimbine on force of contraction and on the cAMP-level were investi- gated. In HR the dose-response curves for the positive inotropic effects (PIE) of IPN and PE were shifted to the right in comparison to NR; thus, the pD_2-value for IPN was significantly decreased from 8.39±0.07(N=8) to 7.99±0.1(N=4), that for PE from 5.44±0.08(N=5) to 4.93±0.08 (N=9). In NR a submaximal effective concentra- tion (EC$_{80}$ for the PIE) of IPN(3×10^{-8}M) increa- sed the cAMP-level after 60sec by about 60%; in HR, however, the same concentration produced only a 25% increase in cAMP. The EC$_{80}$ for the PIE of PE(10^{-5}M) increased in NR the cAMP-level by approximately 35%, but failed to increase it in HR. When used in three times higher concen- trations, however, both agents produced in HR an increase of the cAMP-level comparable with the effects in NR.
From the present results it is concluded that hypothyroidism does not only increase the sen- sitivity of myocardial α-adrenoceptors (Naka- shima et al., Japan.J.Pharmacol. 21, 819, 1971) but in addition reduces the sensitivity of cardiac ß-adrenoceptors. The results confirm the close correlation of the ß-sympathomimetic PIE to the cAMP generating system.

Institute of Pharmacology, University of Essen, Hufelandstrasse 55, D-4300 Essen.

101

ADENYLATE CYCLASE AND SPECIFICITY OF THE HISTAMINE H_2-RECEPTOR IN THE GASTRIC MUCOSA OF THE GUINEA-PIG H.-J. Ruoff

Experimental data indicate that the histamine activated gastric mucosal adenylate cyclase (AC) of the guinea-pig is inhibited by histamine H_1 and H_2-receptor antagonists and the question raises whether the activation of AC occurs via a specific H_2-receptor mechanism as it is known for the histamine stimulated gastric secretion. Receptor specificity of AC-activation and inhibition was tested by selective H_1 (PEA) and H_2 (dimaprit)-receptor agonists and antagonists (mepyramine and cimetidine) in two broken cell preparations (P1 and P2) of the guinea-pig gastric mucosa. P1 consisted of the mucosal homogenate in 25 mM Tris-HCl buffer pH 7.4 containing 1 mM EDTA and 1 mM dithiotreithol, P2 of the 2000·g pellet 3 times resuspended in the homogenisation medium. When P1 was used as enzyme no difference could be detected between the histamine and dimaprit dose response curves. Both compounds (Ka=$5\cdot10^{-6}$ M) actived the basal AC maximally 8-10 fold. PEA (Ka=10^{-4} M) had only a 3-4 fold stimulating action. Maximal activation of AC by PEA and dimaprit was not additive. Cimetidine (10^{-6} M) reduced the histamine or dimaprit stimulated AC by 50 %, whereas mepyramine (10^{-6}M) was ineffective. To achieve the same degree of inhibition with this blocker a concentration of 10^{-3} M was necessary. When P2 was used as enzyme histamine and dimaprit (same Ka as above) activated the basal AC maximally only 5-6 fold. The stimulatory effect of PEA was not reduced. In this preparation the inhibitory profile of cimetidine did not differ from that of mepyramine, i.e. cimetidine (10^{-6} M) was ineffective and a concentration of 10^{-3} M had to be employed to block the histamine activated AC by 50 %. Resuspension of P2 with the supernatant did not restore the original H_2-receptor specificity. The data suggest: AC-activation by histamine is a H_2-receptor mediated process and H_2-receptor specificity is destroyed during the preparation of gastric mucosal membranes.

Pharmakologisches Institut der Universität Tübingen
Wilhelmstrasse 56, D-7400 Tübingen

102

HISTAMINE-SENSITIVE ADENYLATE CYCLASE OF HUMAN GASTRIC MUCOSA: A MODEL FOR H 2 RECEPTOR EXCITATION. B. Simon , W.Schunack,H.Kather,B.Kommerell

Recent studies revealed that human gastric mucosa contains a histamine-sensitive adenylate cyclase which is almost completely localized within the acid-secreting area of the stomach. In an attempt to further characterize the effector system of histamine's action, we compared the effects of H 1 - and H 2-receptor agonists upon the adenylate cyclase in human fundic gastric mucosa.
Stomach tissue was obtained by subtotal gastric resection from patients suffering from peptic ulcer. The adenylate cyclase was assayed in the total homogenate according to SALOMON et al.(Anal.Biochem.54:541,1974).
Basal enzyme activity of Billroth II resection material averaged 0.5 nmol cAMP/mg prot./15 min. The H 2-receptor agonists 4-methyl-histamine , N^{α}-5-dimethyl-histamine and N^{α}-methyl-histamine increased the activity in the fundic mucosa preparation. The degree of stimulation produced by these H 2-agonists did not differ significantly from that generated by histamine up to 1 mM. At this concentration a 2.5-fold increase of enzyme activity was observed. Half maximal stimulation was achieved at H 2 agonist concentrations of about 2o-5o uM. N^{α}-methyl-histamine appears to have a slightly higher affinity to adenylate cyclase than histamine. The H 1-receptor agonists 2-pyridyl-ethylamine, 2-phenyl-histamine and 2-(3-pyridyl)-histamine were much less potent in activating the adenylate cyclase system in fundic mucosa. A small increase of enzyme activity was observed at a H 1-agonist concentrations of 1 mM (about 2o-3o %).
Our results on human fundic adenylate cyclase correlate quite well with data for the H 2-systems and are clearly different from the results on the H 1-receptors.

Gastroenterologische Abteilung der Medizin.Univ.-Klinik, Heidelberg und Pharmazeutisches Institut der Universität Mainz.

103

EFFECT OF METHYLXANTHINES ON EXTRACELLULAR AND INTRACELLULAR 5'-NUCLEOTIDASE ACTIVITY IN ISOLATED FAT CELLS. U. Schwabe

Adenosine is constantly released from isolated fat cells into the incubation medium in quantities that inhibit cyclic AMP accumulation and lipolysis in response to lipolytic hormones. Adenosine is generated from 5'-AMP by a 5'-nucleotidase which is located at the extracellular face of the fat cell plasma membrane (A.C. Newby et al., Biochem. J. 146, 625-633; 1975). Therefore, the effect of several stimulators of cyclic AMP dependent lipolysis on rat fat cell 5'-nucleotidase was studied. 5'-Nucleotidase activity in intact rat fat cells was measured at substrate concentrations of 1 μM 5'-AMP and was linear for 10 min under these conditions. Noradrenaline (3μM) and adenosine deaminase (10 μg/ml) had no effects on the activity of 5'-nucleotidase. The activity was inhibited by theophylline and caffeine and 50 % inhibition was observed at a concentration of 0.5 mM. The inhibition by these methylxanthines occurred also in particulate preparations of fat cells. It was independent from the fat cell concentration in the incubation medium and was not influenced by adenosine up to 100 μM. Other phosphodiesterase inhibitors which are not able to induce lipolysis like papaverine (0,1 mM) and Ro 20-1724 (0,1 mM) had no influence on the 5'-nucleotidase activity. The results indicate that methylxanthines in addition to their effect on cyclic AMP phosphodiesterase may increase cAMP levels and lipolysis in fat cells by inhibiting the adenosine generating enzyme and thereby prevent the antilipolytic control by endogenous adenosine.

Institut für Pharmakologie, Medizinische Hochschule Hannover, Karl-Wiechert-Allee 9, D-3000 Hannover 61

104

DIHYDROCAFFEIC ACID, A METABOLITE OF BIOFLAVONOIDS, AS A COFACTOR OF PROSTAGLANDIN SYNTHETASE J. Baumann, F. v. Bruchhausen, G. Wurm, and R. Hänsel

The influence of dihydrocaffeic acid (I), a main metabolite of bioflavonoids, on prostaglandin synthesis was studied on a preparation of rat renal medulla. In comparison, caffeic acid (II), isoferulic acid (III), protocatechuic acid (IV), vanillic acid (V) and 3(4-hydroxyphenyl)-propionic acid (VI) in equimolar concentrations (10^{-3} M) were tested. When incubated without adrenaline, I, II, and III increased the yield of prostaglandin E from [^{14}C]arachidonic acid by about 100%. IV and V show lower efficacy, whereas VI is nearly without effect. In the investigated system dihydrocaffeic acid can thus substitute adrenaline as cofactor. The half-maximal effective concentration (I_{50}) calculated from the concentration response plot is $7.5 \cdot 10^{-5}$ M. Dihydrocaffeic acid is far more potent than L-tryptophan which, according to T. Miyamoto, N. Ogino, S. Yamamoto, and O. Hayaishi (J. biol. Chem. 251, 2629, 1976) is supposed to be the important cofactor for the conversion of prostaglandin G to prostaglandin H (peroxidase reaction). In the pattern of stepwise formation of prostaglandin E from arachidonic acid the influence of dihydrocaffeic acid is studied in the presence of hematin which enables the fatty acid cyclooxygenase reaction. The site of action of caffeic acid and the question, whether the possible formation of quinonoid structures may be essential for the cofactor function in prostaglandin synthesis are discussed.

Institut für Pharmakologie der Freien Universität Berlin, Thielallee 69/73, D-1000 Berlin 33

105

EFFECT OF CYCLIC NUCLEOTIDE PHOSPHODIESTERASE INHIBITORS ON PROSTAGLANDIN BIOSYNTHESIS   I. Ahnfelt-Rønne and M.P. Magnussen

The xanthine-derivatives theophylline (TPH), caffeine (CAF) theobromine (TBR) and 1-methyl-3-isobutyl-xanthine (MIX) are well-known inhibitors of cyclic nucleotide phosphodiesterase (PDE), and many of their in vivo effects have been attributed to impairment of cyclic AMP hydrolysis (e.g. bronchodilation, diuretic action, effect on heart). It was observed, however, that these drugs are also potent stimulators of prostaglandin synthetase (PGS) from bovine seminal vesicle microsomes (BSVM) in vitro. Papaverine (PAP), a PDE-inhibitor chemically unrelated to xanthine, had no effect on PGS. It was also found that BSVM have high PDE-activity, and dose-response curves were established with the xanthines and PAP in regard to BSVM-PDE inhibition and BSVM-PGS stimulation.

compound	PGS-stim. ED$_{50}$ (mM)	cAMP-PDE inh. IC$_{50}$ (mM)	cGMP-PDE inh. IC$_{50}$ (mM)	L.I. %
PAP	no effect	0.007	0.03	n.d.
MIX	0.93	0.06	0.16	90.4
CAF	1.30	2.40	1.00	99.6
TPH	2.70	2.70	1.40	21.3
TBR	3.00	>5	7.50	32.8

ED$_{50}$: Conc. that stimulate 50% of maximal response with CAF (2.6 times basal activity at 10 mM).
[Cyclic AMP] = [Cyclic GMP] = 10 μM during incubation.
L.I.: Lipophilic index, i.e. % of drug found in CHCl$_3$ after distribution between equal vol. of CHCl$_3$ and 0.1 M K$^+$-phosphate buffer pH 8 (PGS assay buffer).

Since PAP had no effect on PGS, and cyclic AMP and cyclic GMP up to 1 mM were also ineffective, whether alone or in presence of TPH, it is concluded that xanthines stimulate PGS directly, and not via cyclic nucleotides. This effect might also have significance in vivo.

Department of Pharmacology, Leo Pharmaceutical Products, Industriparken 55, DK-2750 Ballerup, Denmark.

106

PROSTAGLANDINS AND CYCLIC AMP IN PROLIFERATING FIBROBLASTS. P.S. Schönhöfer, A. Wasmus and I. Klappstein

Inhibition of prostaglandin (PG) biosynthesis by indometacin (0.01 μM) resulted in enhanced proliferation in L cells which was inhibited by addition of 30 μM PGE$_1$ (D.R.Thomas et al, Exptl.Cell Res.84,40,1974), indicating that PGE$_1$ may play a role in the regulation of cellular proliferation.

In secondary embryonic mouse fibroblasts, addition of 10 μM PGE$_1$ was able to reduce the proliferation rate similar to the effects obtained by Bt$_2$-cAMP. Addition of a phosphodiesterase (PDE) inhibitor did not significantly augment the effect of PGE$_1$. The inhibitory action of PGE$_1$ on cell proliferation was correlated to a rise in intracellular cAMP levels which remained higher than controls for 24-48 hrs after addition. PGE$_1$ plus PDE inhibitor had only moderate effect on intracellular cAMP levels as compared to PGE$_1$ alone, but caused an up to tenfold rise in the extracellular cAMP levels. Thus the inhibitory effect of PGE$_1$ on cell proliferation correlated with the increase in intracellular cAMP levels. Indometacin and prednisolone at concentrations (0.5 μM) which inhibit endogenous PG formation did not cause an increase in cell proliferation. The lack of effect was again reflected in the intracellular cAMP levels which were not reduced by both inhibitors of PG formation.

These findings argue for a compensatory mechanism by which the cells are able to maintain their basal cAMP levels even when endogenous PG levels are decreased.

Institut für Pharmakologie, Medizinische Hochschule Hannover, Karl-Wiechert-Allee 9, D-3000 Hannover 61, GFR

107

INHIBITION OF PROSTAGLANDIN SYNTHETASE BY 2'-/4,5-bis-(4-chlorphenyl)-oxazolyl-(2)-mercapto/-propionic acid (EMD 26 644) IN VITRO AND IN VIVO M. Klockow, H. Nowak

In pharmacological tests and clinical trials 2'-/4,5-bis-(4-chlorphenyl)-oxazolyl-(2)-mercapto/-propionic acid (EMD 26 644) has proved to be an effective nonsteroidal anti-inflammatory agent (NSTA) and an inhibitor of platelet aggregation.
In vitro EMD 26 644 inhibits prostaglandin synthetase, isolated from bovine seminal vesicles (I$_{50}$ = 0.35 μM). Compared with other NSTA e.g. indomethacine (I$_{50}$ = 0.08 μM) and ibuprofen (I$_{50}$ = 10 μM) EMD 26 644 belongs to the group of NSTA with high inhibitory activity against prostaglandin synthetase. Also the production of prostaglandins by aggregating platelets of rat plasma is inhibited by EMD 26 644. In vivo the influence of EMD 26 644 and other NSTA on the increased level of prostaglandins during intraperitoneal inflammation of rats was determined. 10 mg/kg EMD 26 644 decreased significantly the level of prostaglandins in intraperitoneal fluid.

Med. Research Dept., E. Merck, Darmstadt

108

RELEASE OF PROSTAGLANDIN D$_2$ AND THROMBOXANE B$_2$ FROM HUMAN THROMBOCYTES: RADIOIMMUNOLOGICAL DETERMINATION AND MODIFICATION BY DRUGS.
H. Anhut, B.A. Peskar and B.M. Peskar

Radioimmunoassays for prostaglandin D$_2$ (PGD$_2$) and thromboxane B$_2$ (TXB$_2$) were developed. Antisera were obtained from rabbits immunized with the corresponding hapten-bovine serum albumine conjugates. The conjugates were synthesized using N,N'-carbonyldiimidazole as coupling reagent (Axen, Prostaglandins 5, 45, 1974). The radioactive tracer for the TXB$_2$ assay was synthesized by incubation of ^{3}H-arachidonic acid as substrate with washed human thrombocytes as enzyme source. The label for the PGD$_2$ assay was also synthesized from ^{3}H-arachidonic acid using the microsomal fraction of sheep seminal vesicles as enzyme source. Both radioimmunoassays are highly specific and recognize the ring structure and the hydroxyl group at position C$_{15}$ as immunodominant parts of the hapten molecules. The detection limits are 40 pg for TXB$_2$ and 200 pg for PGD$_2$. The radioimmunoassays were used to determine the release of TXB$_2$ and PGD$_2$ from washed human thrombocytes after addition of thrombin. While only small amounts of immunoreactive PGD$_2$ were released in control incubates, the TX synthetase inhibitor imidazole (1.47 mM) increased PGD$_2$ as well as PGF$_{2\alpha}$ and PGE$_2$ release and simultaneously reduced TXB$_2$ release significantly. Indometacin (2.8 μM) abolished both TXB$_2$ and PG release in response to thrombin. The PGD$_2$ found in the incubates could be formed either enzymatically or nonenzymatically by isomerization from its endoperoxide precursor PGH$_2$. The thrombin-induced formation of PGD$_2$ by thrombocytes could be important in view of the potent antiaggregatory activity of PGD$_2$.

Department of Pharmacology and Med. Clin., University of Freiburg, Hermann-Herder-Strasse 5, D 7800 Freiburg i. Br.

109

EFFECTS OF DRUGS ON THE PROSTAGLANDIN RELEASE
FROM MACROPHAGES IN VITRO   K. Brune, M. Glatt
and H. Kälin

Macrophages play a key role in mediating inflammatory reactions.They are believed to fulfil
this function in part by releasing prostaglan-
dins(PG's).These cells can be cultured in vitro
and may be triggered to release PG's by adding
phagocytosable particles (M.Glatt et al.,Agents
and Actions, 7, 321, 1977). Consequently, macrophages in cell culture appear suitable for inve-
vestigating the mechanisms involved in PG release. We found that PG-release from phagocytosing
mouse peritoneal macrophages may be reduced or
enhanced by different drugs. Non-steroidal anti-
inflammatory drugs inhibited PG-release without
influencing phagocytosis. 2-deoxyglucose inhibited both phagocytosis and PG-release.Cytochala-
sin B enhanced PG-release but interfered with
phagocytosis.These results suggest that phagocytosis and PG-release are independent events.How-
ever, transmission electron microscopic analysis
of the cellular events going along with PG-release indicate an alternative interpretation. 2-
deoxyglycose inhibited phagocytosis and preserved the intracellular separation of lysosomes,
endoplasmic reticulum and mitochondria.Secondary
lysosomes were virtually absent in these cells.
By contrast,cytochalasin B induced fusion of different components of the endovesicular system
with the cell membranes and with each other despite inhibition of phagocytosis. This observation suggests that the fusion of lysosomes with
compounds of the endovesicular system may be a
crucial step for the synthesis of PG's.

Department of Pharmacology, Biozentrum, University of Basle, Switzerland.

110

THE EFFECT OF PROSTAGLANDIN E_1 (PGE_1) ON THE PLASMA -
LYMPH BARRIER OF THE HIND LIMB OF RABBITS AND THE AN-
TAGONISTIC EFFECT OF ESCIN AND INDOMETHACIN
M.Rothkopf-Ischebeck

One of the lymph vessels close to the femoral artery
of the hind limb of rabbits was cannulated and the
lymph was collected for periods of 30 min.After infusing 0.9% NaCl solution into a side vessel of the
femoral artery for 90 min either 12.5, 19, 25 or 50
ng/kg/min PGE_1 were infused for a period of 15 min.
Fifteen min after the infusion of 12.5 to 25 ng/kg/
min PGE_1 the lymph flow was increased by 13% to 81% ;
following 50 ng/kg/min PGE_1 a maximum increase of 92%
was evident 45 min after infusion.Approximately 105
min after PGE_1-infusion,lymph flow was no longer in-
creased.Based on a criterion of $\geq$ 50% increase of
lymph flow the ED_{50} 15 min after infusion was 19 ng/
kg/min.At the dose of 50 ng/kg/min side effects such
as diarrhoea,muscle tremor,salivation and increase in
respiration rate were evident.Up to the dose of 25 ng
/kg/min no hemodynamic effects occured.
One hour before PGE_1-infusion escin was injected at
doses of 0.25, 0.50 and 0.80 mg/kg i.v.,whereas indomethacin was injected into the ear vein at doses of
either 10 or 20 mg/kg immediately after the PGE_1 -
infusion of 25 ng/kg/min (ED_{75}).Fortyfive min after
PGE_1-infusion escin decreased the lymph flow by about
45% to 92% and indomethacin by about 49% to 62% in
comparison to control animals.Based on a criterion of
$\geq$ 50% inhibition of the enhanced lymph flow the ED_{50}
of escin was 0.29 mg/kg.
According to these experiments escin and indomethacin
revealed a strong antagonistic effect of the permeability increasing action of PGE_1.Whether escin is a
direct antagonist of PGE_1 cannot be clarified by these
experiments,for PGE_1 was administered exogeneously.

Department of Pharmacology,Dr.Madaus & Co.
D 5 Köln,Ostmerheimerstr. 198

111

PHARMACOLOGICAL ACTIONS OF PROSTACYCLIN (PGI_2)
B.A. Schölkens and U. Weithmann

Prostacyclin (PGI_2), a newly discovered unstable intermediate of arachidonic acid, was injected i.v. in
anaesthetized and conscious animals to test the cardiovascular and respiratory effects. The sodium salt
of PGI_2 was used, synthetized according to Nicolaou
et al. (1977). It relaxed bovine coronary arteries,
whereas rat stomach strip, guinea pig ileum and
uterus were contracted. PGI_2 inhibited arachidonic
acid-induced aggregation (human platelet-rich plasma)
at 9×10^{-9}M (50%) or reversed it. In anaesthetized
normotensive rats, rabbits and dogs PGI_2 in doses between 0.1-1 µg/kg i.v. significantly decreased systemic arterial blood pressure (BP) in a dose dependent
manner. Such a depressor response could also be demonstrated in conscious rats with chronic catheters.
In rats with acute elevation of BP, produced by un-
clamping one renal pedicle which had been occluded
for four hours, i.v. injection of PGI_2 was followed
by a significant fall in BP. Angiotensin II and noradrenaline induced increase of systemic BP was reversed by PGI_2. Pretreatment with phentolamin or propranolol did not influence the fall in BP. In the anaesthetized dog a fall in left ventricular systolic
pressure and an increase in myocardial contractility
with marginal changes in heart rate could be observed. PGI_2 inhibited significantly 5-HT induced
increases in pulmonary resistance and decreases in
lung compliance in a dose dependent manner in anaesthetized cats.

Hoechst AG., D-6230 Frankfurt (Main) 80, Federal
Republic of Germany

112

SULPROSTONE (CP-34,089, ZK 57 671), A PROSTAGLANDIN
E_2 ANALOGUE WITH POTENT ANTIFERTILITY EFFECTS AND
IMPROVED SELECTIVITY FOR UTERINE SMOOTH MUSCLES
O. Loge, E. Schillinger, and W. Losert

PG E_2 and PG $F_{2\alpha}$ stimulate uterine smooth muscles and
can be used for induction of abortion. The therapeutic potential is, however, reduced by their lack
of tissue selectivity which results in a variety of
side-effects.
Sulprostone (S, 16-Phenoxy-ω-tetranor-PG E_2-methyl-
sulfonylamide) showed uterine stimulating activity
comparable with PG E_2, but had little or no effect on
other cell/organ functions. This was demonstrated in
vitro (uterine, intestinal, vascular, tracheal smooth
muscles; platelets; fat cells; PG receptor binding)
as well as in vivo by different organ function tests
including the simultaneous recording of intrauterine
(UP), intestinal, intrapleural, and blood (BP) pressure, heart and respiratory rate, as well as respiratory volume in anaesthetized rabbits. The only substance tested with comparable tissue selectivity was
PG I_2. Wheras S (10 and 50 µg/kg i.v., resp.) almost
exclusively increased UP, PG I_2 (1 and 5 µg/kg i.v.,
resp.) only reduced BP. In contrast to S and PG I_2,
PG E_2 and PG $F_{2\alpha}$ (10 and/or 50 µg/kg i.v., resp.)
influenced all organ functions studied. With the exception of UP, their effects differed qualitatively
or quantitatively.It is suggested that the characteristic pharmacological profile of S results from a
favourable combination of PG E- and PG F-type
properties.

Research Laboratories, Schering AG,
Müllerstraße 170-178, D-1000 Berlin 65

113

CHARACTERIZATION OF CARDIOACTIVE AGENTS USING THE ANALYSIS OF THE VENTRICULAR PRESSURE CURVE DURING ISOVOLUMETRIC CONTRACTION   U. Borchard, K. Greeff and D. Hafner

The rate of rise of ventricular pressure during contraction depends on the myocardial contractile state, the loading conditions and on autoregulation. The characterization of cardioactive agents by measuring peak dP/dt may be contradictory if the diastolic arterial pressure decreases simultaneously. In order to discriminate changes in loading from cardiac inotropy several indices of contractility have been suggested. If arterial diastolic pressure decreases without significant changes in end-diastolic pressure or autoregulation, the inotropic state may be best characterized by the analysis of ventricular pressure during isovolumetric contraction (D.T.Mason, Am. J. Cardiol., 23, 516,1969).
The experiments were performed with cats receiving an infusion of 2 or 1.69 mg/kg · min carticaine or lidocaine and 1 to 10 µg/kg · min sodium nitroprusside (SNP). Left ventricular pressure and LVdP/dt were registered by means of a digital computer and evaluated by an off-line programme. 10 min after infusion of the local anaesthetics, a peak common developed isovolumetric pressure (CPIP) and corresponding values of LVdP/dt were determined, and the ratio LVdP/dt /CPIP was plotted against the logarithm of dose. Reference values of this ratio were found to be ($\pm$ S.E.M.): 102.6 ± 6.0 sec^{-1}(carticaine, n = 7) and 99.3 ± 9.9 sec^{-1} (lidocaine, n = 8). Logarithmic increase in dose brought about a linear decrease in the ratio which after 10 min amounted to ($\pm$ S.E.M.): 46.4 ± 3.9 sec^{-1} (carticaine) and 40.3 ± 4.1 sec^{-1} (lidocaine).The significant decrease of the ratio (P $\leq$ 0.005) after 1 min of infusion of both local anaesthetics indicates a negative inotropic action. SNP, which decreases diastolic arterial pressure up to 40%, did not alter the ratio if the heart rate remained unchanged. This demonstrates that SNP has no influence on cardiac inotropy.

Department of Pharmacology, University of Düsseldorf, Moorenstr. 5, D-4000 Düsseldorf.

114

THE INFLUENCE OF D 600, OUABAIN, AND CALCIUM ON THE POST-REST ADAPTATION IN GUINEA PIG PAPILLARY MUSCLE.   R. Becher

In guinea pig papillary muscle, the force of contraction and the action potentials showed characteristic patterns of adaptation after various periods of rest. These patterns could be influenced by pharmacological agents. After 10 min of rest, the contraction amplitude was small. At 1 Hz the force of contraction increased monotonically to reach pre-rest control values within 3-5 min. The post-rest changes of the action potential duration (a.p.d.) on the other hand were biphasic. Starting from a first action potential which was clearly longer than the pre-rest value, the duration of the consecutive action potentials increased rapidly, reached a maximum, and then declined slowly to the control level. The time course of the post-rest adaptation of the a.p.d. could be described by the sum of two exponential functions, each of which being regarded as a cumulation curve. This suggests the presence of two indepent and opposing processes, one prolonging and the other one shortening the a.p.d.. They were called the lengthening and shortening effect of activation (LEA and SEA, respectively). Two similar opposing processes during activation have been described for the post-rest changes in mechanical activity by KOCH-WESER and BLINKS (1963).

LEA and SEA could be influenced seperately by pharmacological agents. By lowering the extracellular calcium concentration, the influence of SEA was diminished; ouabain (2×10^{-7}M) reduced the effect of LEA; the compound D 600 (1×10^{-6}M), however, shortened the a.p.d. by a process other than SEA.

Department of Pharmacology, University of Kiel, D 23 Kiel, Hospitalstrasse 4-6

115

THE INFLUENCE OF METHOXY-VERAPAMIL (D 600) ON THE FREQUENCY DEPENDENT ACTIVATION OF E-C-COUPLING EFFICIENCY IN GUINEA PIG ATRIA.   E. Ziehm

Two oppositely acting but simultaneously occurring processes are thought to determine the force frequency relationship of cardiac muscle. One process increases the force of contraction presumably due to an enhanced availability of activating Ca^{++}. A second one reduces the force, probably reflecting an inadequate rebinding of Ca^{++} during the shortened beat interval to those structures, from which Ca becomes ionized upon depolarization. The first process can seperately be evaluated by the method described by K.A.P. Edman and M. Johannsson (J. Phys. Lon. 254, 565 1976). The influence on this process of ouabain and methoxy-verapamil was studied in isolated left auricles of guinea pig. The muscles were driven at 1 Hz during the control period, thereafter stimulated at different frequencies (0.5 - 4 Hz) for a constant number of beats (priming period) and again stimulated with 1 Hz. The force of the first contraction (test contraction) following the priming period was evaluated. The force of the test contraction increased with the frequency applied during the priming period. The relation between the force of the test contraction and the priming frequency obeyed a hyperbolic function. Under control conditions the half maximal effect was achieved by a frequency of 2.2 ± 0.2 Hz, in presence of ouabain (3×10^{-7}M) at about 1.2 Hz and with methoxy verapamil (1×10^{-7}M) at 3.1 ± 0.1 Hz. The calculated maximum of this process was not altered by the drugs. It is concluded that ouabain facilitates the development of the "Treppe"-phenomenon, whereas in the presence of methoxy-verapamil higher stimulation rates are required to achieve a comparable increase in force of contraction. The same conclusion was drawn from the influence of both drugs on the relation between the force of the post rest contraction and the duration of rest (T. Ziegler and E. Ziehm Naunyn-Schmiedeberg's Arch. Pharmacol. 297, 91 1977).

Department of Pharmacology, University of Kiel, D 23 Kiel, Hospitalstrasse 4 - 6

116

The Effect Of Adriamycin On The Isometric Contraction Of Guinea-Pig Papillary Muscle. Muscle mechanics and Electrophysiology. B. Höfling and H.-D. Bolte

Previous studies pointed out that severe cardiotoxic side effects restrict the use of Adriamycin (A) as an effective cancer therapeutic agent. In order to study acute and chronic A-effects on muscle mechanics and electrophysiological properties, experiments were done in isolated papillary muscles from guinea-pig under conditions of isometric contraction. Action potential was measured by use of glass micro-electrodes. In 28 muscles of not pretreated animals maximum isometric tension development (T_{max}) was reduced by $15.8\pm7.5\%$ following an increasing A-concentration (2-80 ug/ml). Maximum rate of tension development (dT/dt_{max}) decreased by $14.7\pm5.9\%$. Maximally effective concentration: 8-10 ug/ml. Electrophysiological properties such as resting potential, action potential, overshoot,upstroke velocity and duration of action pot. did not change. After pretreatment with A for 1-4 courses (course: 3 days 1mg/kg A; 4 days interval) maximum isometric tension development/cross sectional area and further acute A-effect were reduced variably, when compared to untreated animals. However, the cardiotoxic effect of A-pretreatment became more evident and reproducable after addition of epinephrine (12 ug/ml). Whereas T_{max} of muscles from untreated animals increased by about 100% there was a diminuation of response in muscles of pretreated animals. This diminuation could be correlated with duration and dose of A-pretreatment. In summary and conclusion: 1.Both, acute and chron, A-effects can be observed. 2.Musclemech. changes are not due to changes in electrical membrane properties or to change in exciting-contraction coupling. 3.Cardiotoxic effect (clinically often sudden, irreversible congestive heart failure) may be detected most sensitive by (clinical) use of a stimulatory test.

Deparment of Medicine I, Klinikum Großhadern, University of Munich, 8 München 70, Marchioninistr. 15

117

THE EFFECT OF ANEMONIA SULCATA TOXIN ATX II ON POST-REST ADAPTATION IN GUINEA PIG PAPILLARY MUSCLE.
P. Döderlein

In isolated papillary muscle of the guinea pig electrical and mechanical activity were recorded at a stimulation rate of 1/s. After a long period of rest (10 min) the contraction amplitude showed a monotonous adaptation to pre-rest controls whereas the time course of the changes in action potential duration (a.p.d.) was biphasic, i.e. after a rapid prolongation, a transient maximum was reached, which was followed by a much slower shortening in a.p.d. to control values.

In normal Tyrode solution, ATX II (2×10^{-8} M) caused a steady state prolongation of the a.p.d. from 233 ± 8 to 275 ± 23 ms, and a prolongation of the transient maximum in post-rest a.p.d. from 295 ± 8 to 481 ± 60 ms. With partial depolarization in K^+-rich medium the time course of post-rest adaptation of the a.p.d. became essentially monotonic. Under this condition ATX II was ineffective in prolonging the a.p.d. during equilibrium as well as during adaptation. When the extracellular Na^+- concentration was lowered to 70 mM, the a.p.d. was found to be 216 ± 16 ms. The transient maximum during post-rest adaptation of the a.p.d. reached 318 ± 31 ms. Extremely long action potentials, i.e. maximal values of 703 ± 248 ms, were recorded during post-rest adaptation in the presence of 2×10^{-8} M ATX II with 70 mM Na^+.

These findings suggest that the fast sodium channels may play an important role in post-rest adaptation phenomena.

Department of Pharmacology, University of Kiel, D 23 Kiel, Hospitalstrasse 4-6

119

THE EFFECT OF ACETYLCHOLINE AND cGMP ON SLOW RESPONSE ACTION POTENTIAL AND CONTRACTILE FORCE IN MAMMALIAN ATRIAL MYOCARDIUM
M. Kohlhardt and K. Haap

In isolated myocardium from the left atrium of guinea pigs, the effect of acetylcholine (ACh) and 8-Br-cGMP on the slow response action potential and on contractile force was studied. ACh reduced upstroke velocity and overshoot and abbreviated action potential duration. Though the sensitivity towards ACh ($1.65 \cdot 10^{-8}$ M - $5.5 \cdot 10^{-6}$ M) widely differed, the decline of upstroke velocity was accompanied by similar quantitative changes of contractile force. The same depression of the slow response action potential was caused by 8-Br-cGMP ($6 \cdot 10^{-4}$ M). Upstroke velocity was diminished by 12 - 58 % and isometric contractile force by 8 - 53 %. The β-adrenergic compound isoproterenol abolished the inhibitory effects of 8-Br-cGMP. However, the absolute values of upstroke velocity, overshoot, and contractile force reached in the presence of isoproterenol were lower when the preparation had been pretreated with 8-Br-cGMP. These results indicate that cGMP might mediate the ACh effect on the surface membrane. The decline of upstroke velocity of the atrial slow response action potential suggests that 8-Br-cGMP could exert an inhibitory action on the Ca-carried slow inward current.

Physiological Institute, University of Freiburg, Hermann-Herder-Str.7, D-78 Freiburg, Fed.Rep.

118

DEXAMETHASONE-INDUCED TOLERANCE TO CARDIAC ANOXIA: RÔLE OF MUSCLE GLYCOGEN LEVELS AND SERUM INSULIN
K. Schlossmann, R. Towart

Dexamethasone pretreatment of rats produces a marked tolerance to cardiac anoxia in in vitro experiments (Towart and Schlossmann, Naunyn Schmiedebergs Arch. Pharmacol. 297, R 24, 1977). After acute administration (8 mg/kg i.m. dexamethasone) the tolerance to anoxia develops within 3 to 6 h. It can be shown that this tolerance to anoxia is due to an increased concentration of glycogen, which acts as an anaerobic energy reserve, in the heart muscle. The concentration of glycogen increases from the 3rd h after application and reaches the maximum 12 h after application.
To investigate the mechanism of action of this phenomenon we have in addition measured the metabolic substrates in blood, liver and skeletal muscle. Dexamethasone 8 mg/kg i.m. increased the glycogen concentration of liver and of skeletal muscle significantly from 6 h after administration. Investigation of the serum levels of insulin also showed an increase from the 6th h after dexamethasone application in comparison to saline-treated control animals.
Our results show that the dexamethasone induced increase in heart glycogen concentration which is responsible for the increased tolerance to anoxia of this organ is probably produced by the considerable increase in serum insulin levels and can be considered as an indirect consequence of the catabolic and gluconeogenetic effects of dexamethasone.

Institut für Pharmakologie der BAYER AG, D 5600 Wuppertal 1, Postfach 101709

120

THE EFFECT OF ANEMONIA SULCATA TOXIN (ATX II) ON THE CALCIUM CONTENT AND ITS EXCHANGEABILITY IN SPONTANEOUSLY BEATING ATRIA OF THE GUINEA PIG
J. Preuner and U. Ravens

In heart muscle the Anemonia sulcata toxin ATX II has a pronounced positive inotropic effect without a significant change in time-to-peak tension. In order to elucidate whether the positive inotropic effect is due to changes in the calcium turnover we determined the total tissue calcium content and the uptake of ^{45}Ca in spontaneously beating atria of the guinea pig. Two concentrations of ATX II were used: 1×10^{-8} M ATX II augmented contractile force by 45%, whereas 1×10^{-7} M ATX II induced arrhythmia and contracture. With 1.2 mM Ca^{++} in the incubation medium the average total tissue calcium amounted to 270 nequ./100 mg w.w.; after 60 min 68% of the total tissue content had exchanged with ^{45}Ca. With 1×10^{-8} M ATX II, neither total tissue calcium nor ^{45}Ca content could be distinguished from the controls. Under these conditions the spontaneous beat frequency remained constant. In the presence of pentobarbital (2×10^{-4} M), a condition under which the exchangeable Ca-fraction was reduced by 30%, no restoration to control levels could be induced by ATX II (1×10^{-8} M) although the negative inotropic effect was reversed. Even a positive inotropic effect could be observed with both pentobarbital and ATX II. In contrast to the action of cardiac glycosides the positive inotropic effect of ATX II cannot be explained by a measurable change in the calcium turnover.
After 90 min of exposure to 1×10^{-7} M ATX II, the total tissue calcium increased to 460 nequ./100 mg w.w.. Simultaneously the ^{45}Ca uptake was markedly depressed. Since the total tissue calcium content increased in spite of the reduced uptake of ^{45}Ca, it is concluded, that the Ca-efflux was reduced to an even greater extent.

Department of Pharmacology, University of Kiel, D 23 Kiel Hospitalstrasse 4 - 6

121

ON THE RATE OF ONSET AND DECLINE OF THE EFFECTS OF
A TERTIARY AND QUARTERNARY CHOLINOMIMETIC DRUG
ON THE CONTRACTILE FORCE AND THE ACTION POTENTIALS
OF GUINEA PIG ATRIA   C. Kücükhüseyin, and A. Ziegler

The rates of the negative inotropic action of carbachol and norarecoline in isolated left guinea pig auricles differ remarkably. The
onset of action as well as the offset upon washout of the drugs
occur more rapidly in the case of carbachol. The same dissociation
was observed when the time courses of the changes of the action
potential duration were studied. The time course of restitution of
the contractile force after removal of the drugs could be influenced
by the experimental conditions. Upon prolonging the period of
exposure to carbachol, the restitution of the contractile force was
accelerated. On the other hand, a prolonged contact with norarecoline slowed the restitution. Part of the observed differences
may be due to the distribution pattern of the drugs. In contrast to
the quarternary carbachol, norarecoline will penetrate the plasma-
lemma and slowly accumulates within the tissue. Thus the time
course of the changes of the norarecoline concentration in the
extracellular space and in vicinity of the muscarinic receptors is
influenced by the slow cellular uptake and release of this drug. In
the case of carbachol, the clearance of the extracellular space
should be independent of the duration of the preceeding exposure.
It is assumed that the enhanced rate of restitution after an extended
exposure to carbachol unveils changes in the calcium distribution
within the cell. This assumption is supported by experiments without pharmacological agents. For example, when the stimulation
frequency was changed to 3 Hz following different periods of low
frequency excitation comparable time courses of the adaptation
to the higher contractility level were observed.

Department of Pharmacology, University of Kiel, D 23 Kiel,
Hospitalstrasse 4 - 6

122

THE POSITIVE INOTROPIC EFFECT OF PHENYLEPHRINE
IN BOVINE CARDIAC MUSCLE   R. Brückner

The effect of phenylephrine (Phe) on the shape of
the isometric contraction curve was studied in
electrically driven (0.3 Hz) trabeculae excised
from the right ventricles of cow hearts. The Phe-
induced positive inotropic effect (PIE) began at
0.1 μM and reached its maximum (225% of control)
at 100 μM. Propranolol, 1 μM, decreased the maximal PIE of Phe by about 30%. In the presence of
propranolol (1 μM) plus phentolamine (5 μM), the
concentration-response curve for the PIE of Phe
was shifted by about 2 log units to the right.
In the presence of propranolol, the PIE of Phe
was accompanied not only by a significant increase in the rate of force development (RFD;
198% of control at 100 μM) but also by a significant increase in time to peak tension (TPT; 110%
of control at 100 μM).
Previous studies have provided evidence that the
PIE of ß- and α- adrenoceptor agonists is caused
by two different mechanisms, a c-AMP-dependent
and a c-AMP-independent one (see Osnes and Øye,
Adv. Cycl. Nucleot. Res. 5, 415, 1975). The former effect is generally accepted to be characterized by a decrease in TPT. The present observation that the α-adrenoceptor mediated PIE of
Phe was accompanied by an increase in TPT indicates that there are also qualitative differences between these two responses.

Abteilung III (Biochemische Pharmakologie), Institut für Pharmakologie und Toxikologie, Medizinische Hochschule Hannover, Karl-Wiechert-
Allee 9, D 3000 Hannover 61

123

POTASSIUM INDUCED LOSS OF THE EARLY COMPONENT
OF MYOCARDIAL CONTRACTION IN PRESENCE OF NOR-
ADRENALINE
Seibel, K. and M. Reiter

In the presence of noradrenaline, the isometric
contraction of the guinea-pig papillary muscle
is composed of two components, an early one
which is frequency-dependent, and a late one
which is fully developed in the rested-state
contraction (see Seibel et al. Naunyn-Schmiedeberg's Arch. Pharmacol. 294, R 19, 1976).
We now found that an increase in $[K]_o$ from 8 to
20 mM abolished the early component but not the
late one (0.2 Hz, 3 x 10^{-6}M noradrenaline). This
effect of K was not caused by an inactivation of
the initial Na current of excitation, since the
inhibition of this current by 60 μM tetrodotoxin
at 8 mM K was without influence upon both contraction components. The effect of K on the early
component resulted from an acceleration of its
decay during the stimulation interval. This was
established by test beats elicited at different
intervals (600 msec to several min) after cessation of stimulation. The steepness of the ascending limb of the early component declined to 30%
within 60, 15 and 2.4 sec at 4 mM, 8 mM and 16
mM $[K]_o$, respectively.
It is concluded that noradrenaline augments the
frequency-dependent (early) component of contraction by increasing the amount of releasable Ca
in a cellular store during activity and augments
the frequency-independent (late) component by
increasing the accumulation of Ca in a second
store during rest. An elevation of $[K]_o$ acceler-
ates the loss of Ca solely from the store responsible for the early component.
Institut für Pharmakologie und Toxikologie der
Technischen Universität München, Biedersteiner
Strasse 29, D-8000 München 40, Bundesrepublik
Deutschland

124

A SECOND STEREOSPECIFIC EFFECT OF PROPRANOLOL ON
THE ISOMETRIC CONTRACTION OF VENTRICULAR MYO-
CARDIUM IN THE PRESENCE OF CATECHOLAMINES.

F. Ebner

The influence of (+)- and (+)-propranolol (4 x
10^{-8} - 10^{-5} M) on the isometric contraction of
the guinea-pig papillary muscle was studied in
presence of (-)-noradrenaline at 3.2 mM Ca^{++},
5.9 mM K^+, 1 Hz stimulation frequency, 35° C.
Propranolol, in addition to its stereospecific
reduction of the inotropic potency of noradrenaline, increased the maximal contraction velocity obtained by the catecholamine (i.e., the klinotropic efficacy). The racemate of propranolol
was 10 times more potent than the dextro isomer
in enhancing the klinotropic maximum of noradrenaline. This supramaximal effect was significantly (p < 0.001) correlated with a decrease
of the accelerating effect of noradrenaline on
relaxation.
The maximal klinotropic effect of (+)-isoprena-
line was enhanced to a similar extent by (+)-
propranolol as that of noradrenaline.
Practolol (1 - 3 x 10^{-5} M) reduced the inotropic
potency of noradrenaline without affecting its
klinotropic maximum.
It is concluded that propranolol as a lipophilic
compound intracellularly inhibits the activating
influence of catecholamines on calcium sequestra-
tion, thereby increasing maximal velocity of contraction.

Institut für Pharmakologie und Toxikologie der
Technischen Universität München, Biedersteiner
Strasse 29, D-8000 München 40, Bundesrepublik
Deutschland

125

FREQUENCY-FORCE RELATIONSHIP AND THE CYCLIC AMP SYSTEM - FUNCTIONAL INVESTIGATIONS IN GUINEA-PIG ATRIA   H.J. Mensing

Considerations of the literature and personal experience suggest that there is more than one mechanism in mammalian atrial myocardium contributing to the positive inotropic effect of a activation (PIEA; J.R.Blinks and J.Koch-Weser, J.Pharmacol.$\underline{134}$,373,1961): besides ionic mechanisms, probably involving accumulation of Ca^{2+} at its release site(s), rate-dependent enzymatic mechanisms controlling ion fluxes are proposed. The activity of sarcolemmal enzymes is considered to be principally subject to modification by the membrane potential. With regard to the cAMP system, adenylate cyclase is certainly a candidate. However, stronger arguments favour cAMP-regulated protein kinase as a key enzyme, being activated by each depolarization: cumulation of PIEA would correlate with increased phosphorylation of a sarcolemmal protein ("slow channel"?); decay of PIEA with cleavage of protein phosphates by a phosphoprotein phosphatase, together with a redistribution of ions.
Experimental: In a special two-chamber bath, 4 ml of a modified KH-medium (mM: Ca^{2+} 1, Mg^{2+} 0.6, dextrose 15; pH 7.4 at 32°C) were rapidly recirculated past left and right atria of young guinea pigs. Left atria were stimulated at 1 Hz with occasional (a) step decreases and (b) periods with frequency slowly changing in the range 0.006 - 1.5 Hz, using a new method for the direct registration of frequency-force loops (see D.Hilgemann et al., Experientia $\underline{33}$,1629, 1977). PIEA disappeared after about a day, and eupaverine, a potent PDE inhibitor, lost its positive inotropic effect. PIEA could be restored with either dibutyryl-cAMP ($EC_{50} \approx$ 3 mM) or orciprenaline, acting similarly: positive inotropy was distinct at 0.006 Hz, and increased considerably in proportion to the stimulation rate, yielding loops not unlike the initial controls. By comparison, ouabain or raised Ca^{2+} clearly acted differently: there were greater force increments at low frequencies, and little further increase, or even a decrease, at higher rates, depending on agent, concentration, and time after isolation of the atria.
Pharmakologisches Institut, D 7400 Tübingen, Wilhelmstr. 56

126

MYOCARDIAL PHOSPHODIESTERASE ACTIVITY IN DIFFERENT MAMMA-LIAN SPECIES   W. Schmitz and E. Kruse

Theophylline (Theo) has been shown to increase myocardial c-AMP in guinea-pig left auricles (Heitmann et al., Arch. Pharmacol. $\underline{293}$, R 96, 1976) but not in atria from reserpine-pretreated rats (Martinez and McNeill, Can. J. Physiol. Pharmacol. $\underline{55}$, 98, 1977). These conflicting results might be due to species differences in phosphodiesterase (PDE) activity. Therefore, we determined PDE activity in different cardiac muscle preparations isolated from guinea pigs and rats. The results (mean PDE activity in pmoles c-AMP hydrolized/ mg protein x min; N = 5-7; substrate concentration 1 μM) are summarized in the Table.

	Left auricle	Right auricle	Left ventricle	Right ventricle
Rat	273.4	298.2	170.0	163.9
Guinea pig	884.3	790.4	943.8	903.9

It is evident that PDE activity in guinea-pig heart preparations was about 3-5 fold higher than PDE activity in rat hearts (p< 0.001 in all cases). Left auricles (LA) were used to determine K_m values and the effects of Theo to inhibit PDE activity. K_m values were the same in LA from guinea pigs and rats (0.45 μM). The IC_{50} for Theo (200 μM) as well as the K_i values (180 μM) were also the same in both preparations.
The results indicate that the differences in the effects of Theo on the c-AMP levels in guinea-pig and rat atrial preparations might indeed be due to species differences in basal PDE activity. It appears likely that the physiological role of PDE may be of different importance in different heart preparations.

Abteilung III (Biochemische Pharmakologie), Institut für Pharmakologie und Toxikologie, Medizinische Hochschule Hannover, Karl-Wiechert-Allee 9, D 3000 Hannover 61

127

EFFECTS OF MAGNESIUM ASPARTATE HYDROCHLORIDE (Mg-Asp.-HCl) ON THE ADRENENERGIC CARDIOPATHY AGGRAVATED BY EPHEDRINE R.Jacob and H.G.Classen

Following treatment with 9-alpha-fluorocortisol (1.5 mg s.c.once daily) and adrenaline (1oo ug and 2oo ug s.c.twice daily, on days 3 and 4), rats (♀,83 to 1oo g) receiving high adrenaline dose exhibited 2o % necroses in the presence of significantly increased myocardial Ca and Na as well as K and Mg increase. Injections of ephedrine (5 mg.s.c., twice daily, on days 3 and 4) caused an increase in heart dry weight, raising the incidence of necroses to 5o % and 61.5% after 1oo ug and 2oo ug adrenaline, enhancing Ca and Na influx and lowering Mg content. Significant derease in K was only seen after high dose of adrenaline.

Administration of Mg-Asp.-HCl (25o and 5oo mg. Mg^{++}/kg.p.o., twice daily) prevented increase in heart dry weight and reduced the incidence of necroses by 4o % and 18 %, The disturbed myocardial electrolyte content was favourably influenced only by 25o mg.Mg^{++}/kg. The unfavourable electrolyte distribution seen after 5oo mg Mg^{++}/kg is attributed to the inhibitory effect of the very high aspartate concentration on Na^+-K^+-ATPase.

Dep. of Nutrition, Pharmacology and Toxicology, University of Hohenheim, D-7ooo Stuttgart 7o, Fruwirthstrasse 14

128

DIFFERENCES IN SUSCEPTIBILITY TO PEPTIDES BE-TWEEN HEART AND VAS DEFERENS OF THE GUINEA PIG H. Iven, E. Kampmann, R. Pursche and G. Zetler

The following peptides were inactive in the non-stimulated isolated vas deferens but increased the twitch due to field stimulation in a dose-dependent manner (mean pD_2 values): angiotensin II amide (A II: 8.1), substance P (SP: 7.8), bradykinin (B: 7.1). The same effects of acetylcholine (6.4) and carbachol (6.5) were antagonized by atropine (pA_2 8.0), but the peptide effects were resistant. The specific A II antagonist sar^1-ala^8-A II left the twitch response unchanged and antagonized competitively (pA_2 7.52) the twitch-enhancing effect of A II but not that of SP and B.
In the guinea-pig papillary muscle, driven at 1 and 3 Hz, neither SP nor B, A II, physalaemin, and met-enkephalin had any effect on action potential parameters or contractility (concentrations 10 - 1000 ng/ml). In the directly stimulated (1/sec) atrium, weak positive inotropic effects were caused by B (pD_2 7.2) but not by SP and A II. Maximum increases in contractility were only 20% of those due to noradrenaline. During field stimulation, SP remained inactive; A II (10 - 30 ng/ml) and B caused weak positive inotropic responses. The effects of B (pD_2 7.08) were by 50% larger than those in the directly stimulated atria.
Conclusions: the muscular tissue of the guinea-pig vas and heart has only low or missing susceptibility to the peptides under investigation: receptors for B, SP and A II are present in the noradrenergic system of the vas but those of SP are missing in that of the atrium.

Abteilung für Pharmakologie, Medizinische Hochschule, Ratzeburger Allee 160, D-2400 Lübeck

129

INHIBITION OF CARDIAC CA⁺⁺ – DEPENDENT MYO-FIBRILLAR ATP-ASE BY ACETALDEHYDE

E. Fassold, W. G. Nayler, W. R. Kukovetz

The effect of acetaldehyde (A), the hepatic metabolite of e-thanol, on cardiac function was investigated on the subcel-lular level. Ca^{++}-dependent enzyme activities of isolated sarcoplasmic reticulum-rich microsomal (SR), mitochondri-al and myofibrillar fractions (guinea-pig hearts) were exa-mined. The concentrations of A used, 0, 02–0,2 mM, have been reported (Majchrowicz and Mendelson, Science 168, 1100, 1970) to occur in human plasma after repeated ethanol in-gestion. The suspended intracellular proteins, layered by 0. 5 ml paraffin to prevent evaporation, were preincubated with A 30–120 min at either 25 or 30°C. These concentra-tions failed to alter Ca^{++}-accumulating (binding and up-take) and ATPase activities of SR and mitochondrial Ca^{++}-uptake. They dose-dependently did, however, inhibit Ca^{++}-dependent and total myofibrillar ATPase but stimulated Ca^{++}-independent (Mg^{++}-dependent) myofibrillar ATPase. The inhibition of Ca^{++}-dependent ATPase could neither be removed by washing nor by increasing the Ca^{++}-concen-tration in the medium. Kinetic studies with varying ATP-concentrations in the presence of 0.2 mM A showed the in-hibition to be competitive. 0. 02–100 mM ethanol had no di-rect effect on myofibrillar ATPase activity. Ca^{++}-binding and uptake by SR are unaffected by these ethanol-concen-trations (Swartz et al., Biochem. Pharmacol. 23, 2369, 1974).

The results indicate an independent, chronic, toxic effect of A on the contraction-apparatus of heart muscle fibres and suggest that it is at least partly responsible for the observed pump dysfunction under acute and longterm alco-hol intake.

Inst. f. Pharmakodyn. u. Tox., Univ. Graz, A-8010, Univ. Pl. 2

130

AFFINITY PARTITIONING OF PLASMAMEMBRANE VESICLES ON DIGOXIN MODIFIED SEPHAROSE

H. Walter

In order to study the interaction of cardiac glycosides with Na^+, K^+-ATPase, plasmamembrane vesicles were isolated from sarcolemm of cardiac muscle (Walter H., Eur. J. Biochem. 58, 595 (1975); Walter H. and Bader H., Eur. J. Biochem. accepted for publication).
The vesicular enzyme was extracted by NaJ and purified by a two-step gradient centrifugation procedure. It exhibits a sensitivity for ouabain of ~90% with respect to ATP-splitting and ~70% with phosphorylation. This shows that a tight glycoside-enzyme-complex is formed during the reaction. In order to study sidedness of this complex, membrane-impermeable polymer-bound digoxin was synthesized. Digoxin was oxidized by JO_4^- to give rise to aldehydes in the terminal digitoxose. This digoxin was coupled to diamine-modified sepharose 6B. Since the final product could be washed with 40% ethanol extensively without loss of the digoxin group, it was concluded that the cardiac glycoside was co-valently bound forming an azomethin.
When membranefragments of sarcolemm were equi-librated with the modified sepharose, less than 5% of the enzyme remained unbound in the super-natant. The addition of an excess of ouabain displaced the bound enzyme to about 10%. However, when intact sarcolemmal vesicles were equilibrated with the sepharose, 20% of the enzyme remained unbound. This result can be seen in context with the observation that about 20 to 30% of the intact vesicles are inside-out, with the ouabain binding site facing the interior.

Department of Pharmacology and Toxicology
University of Ulm, Oberer Eselsberg, 79 Ulm

131

INFLUENCE OF MONOVALENT CATIONS ON THE Ca²⁺-ATPase OF CARDIAC SARCOPLASMIC RETICULUM AND ITS SIGNIFICANS OF THE POSITIVE INOTROP EFFECT OF CARDIAC GLYCOSIDES.

R. Wierichs.

The influence of Na^+ and K^+ on the Ca^{2+}-ATPase of cardiac sarcoplasmic reticulum of pig heart was tested. When 140 mM K^+ was present, the activity of the Ca^{2+}-ATPase was about 20 % higher than in the presence of 140 mM Na^+. This is similar to our results obtained with the Ca^{2+} ATPase of human red blood cell membranes. (Wierichs and Bader, Naunyn-Schmiedeberg's Arch. Pharmacol. 293: Abstr. 170, 1976). Replacing K^+ step by step by Na^+, at constant total monova-lent cation concentrations the Ca^{2+}-ATPase activity was highest when the ration of K^+:Na^+ was 9:1. Decreasing this ration the activity de-creased continuously.
Under therapeutical concentrations of cardiac glycosides the intracellular Na^+ during the action potential is for a prolonged time higher than under normal conditions. (Akera et al., J. Pharm. Exp. Ther. 199: 287, 1976). It is presum-able that thereby the Ca^{2+}-ATPase of the cardiac sarcoplasmic reticulum is partly inhibited. This could be the missing link between the inhibition of the (Na^+ + K^+)-ATPase and the positive ino-trop effect of cardiac glycosides.

Abteilung Pharmakologie und Toxikologie
Universität Ulm, Oberer Eselsberg,
7900 ulm.

132

INFLUENCE OF THE Na-K-ATPase ACTIVITY UPON THE KINE-TICS OF OUABAIN BINDING TO CARDIAC TISSUE

F. Busse, H. Lüllmann, and T. Peters

Rate and degree of ouabain binding to isolated guinea pig atrial muscle depend on 1.) the concentration of the drug applied to the incubation medium, and 2.) the contraction frequency of the pre-parations. Either an increase of the drug concentration at a constant beat frequency or an increase of the beat frequency at a constant drug concentration enhances the rate of binding and the amount of ouabain bound at equilibrium conditions. The data may be explained as follows: 1.) At a given beat frequency and therewith a constant sodium load the ATPase-activity required for Na extrusion remains constant. This also implies that a constant concentration of that particular conformation exists, which is able to bind cardiac gly-cosides. Under this condition the binding kinetics of ouabain are solely governed by the drug concentration in the medium. 2.) At a given concentration of ouabain in the bath but a different fre-quency of contraction the Na-load and the ATPase-activity varies. Hence, the concentration of digitalis binding conformations is determined by the frequency. Under this condition the binding kinetics of ouabain in cardiac tissue appear to be determined by the frequency of contraction. At different beat frequencies differ-ent proportions of the total amount of ATPase molecules are requi-red for the maintenance of Na-K-homeostasis. It is only the frac-tion which is not involved in the ion transport that can be occu-pied by ouabain without an impairment of the homeostasis. That portion of the ATPase which is not required for the maintenance of the homeostasis is believed to mediate the inotropic response upon occupation by cardiac glycosides. This may explain the observation that a given concentration of cardiac glycosides may act positive inotropic at low frequencies of contraction but toxic at higher beat frequencies.

Department of Pharmacology, University of Kiel, D 23 Kiel,
Hospitalstrasse 4 - 6

133

KINETICS OF CHANGES IN K^+-, Na^+- AND Ca^{2+}-CONTENT IN HEART TISSUE IN THE PRESENCE OF CARDIAC GLYCOSIDES. E. Noack, J. Felgenträger and B. Zettner.

It is generally agreed now that cardiac glycosides (CG) specifically react with the Na^+-, K^+-ATPase of the cardiac cell membrane, and it is supposed that such interaction is responsible for the toxic as well as the positive inotropic effect of CG on the heart. If so, it may be expected that the interaction, which may provoke an activation or inhibition of the enzyme, causes intracellular responses in the K^+- and Na^+-balance. In the literature there are, however, very contradictory results concerning changes in the myocardial K^+- and Na^+-content. We, therefore, studied the influence of ouabain (0.1 and 0.2 µM) and digitoxigenin (0.6 µM) in isolated left guinea-pig atria. 3, 5, 10, 15 and 30 min after the addition of the drug, the isometric contraction force, the K^+-, Na^+-, Ca^{2+}-content and the ^{45}Ca-exchange were estimated considering the individual atrial extracellular space volume. In the presence of positive inotropic CG-concentrations, a transient but significant increase of the cellular K^+-content (by 8 to 16%) and corresponding decrease of the Na^+-content (by 20 to 23%) was found 3 to 5 min after the addition. The cellular Ca^{2+}-content significantly decreased by 20 to 30% after 15 min of incubation. If the development of the contraction force was experimentally postponed by lowering the extracellular calcium to 0.9 mM, the maximum of the described K^+- and Na^+-effects was also shifted to longer incubation times. Since isoproterenol (1.8×10^{-8} M) did not show comparable electrolyte changes, the effect is considered to be CG-specific.

Pharmakologisches Institut, Universität Düsseldorf, Moorenstr. 5, 4000 Düsseldorf.

134

EFFECTS OF SPECIFIC 3-H-OUABAIN BINDING TO THE CARDIAC GLYCOSIDE RECEPTOR ON (Na^++K^+)-ATPase ACTIVITY AND ON FORCE OF CONTRACTION IN RAT HEART. G. Philipp, E. Erdmann, and H. Scholz

The exact mechanism of action of cardiac glycosides (CG) is not known. Several investigations have revealed that upon binding of CG to a specific membrane-bound receptor the also membrane-bound $(Na^+ + K^+)$-ATPase is inhibited. This inhibition is supposed to be necessary for the positive inotropic effect of CG. This hypothesis is not unchallenged. We therefore measured at identical conditions in rat heart preparations: 3-H-ouabain binding to isolated cell membranes and to electrically stimulated contracting ventricular strips (ouabain concentration 10^{-9}-10^{-4}M), $(Na^+ + K^+)$-ATPase activity, and contractile force. The time courses of the CG-effects were recorded, too.
Rat heart contains 0.66×10^{14}CG-receptors/g wet weight or 660/µm². Receptors in isolated cell membranes and contracting muscle have a rather high affinity for ouabain, the dissociation constants being 1-3×10^{-7}M(i.e. that free ouabain concentration where 50% of receptors have bound CG-molecules). Half maximal positive inotropic effect occurred at 3×10^{-7}M. Half maximal inhibition of $(Na^+ + K^+)$-ATPase, however, was determined at 4×10^{-5}M. At concentrations where there was ouabain binding to the specific receptors and increased force of contraction, we could not find ATPase inhibited.
Thus, inhibition of $(Na^+ + K^+)$-ATPase in rat heart seems unlikely to be necessary for the positive inotropic effect of CG.

Medizinische Klinik I der Universität München, Klinikum Großhadern, D-8000 München 70, and Institut für Pharmakologie, Medizinische Hochschule Hannover, D-3000 Hannover 61, Germany.

135

PHARMACOKINETICS OF TRITIATED PENTA-ACETYL-GITOXIN IN GUINEA PIGS   G. Haeger and D. Proppe

After single intravenous and oral administrations (i.a., o.a.) of ^{3}H penta-acetyl-gitoxin (0.27 mg/kg, 12 uCi/mg) the elimination of tritium from the blood, its urinary, fecal and biliary excretion as well as tissue to protein-free plasma ratio (T/M), partition coefficient (PC) between $CHCl_3$ and the tissues and plasma, and change in protein binding were investigated in guinea pigs. 1) The overall plasma tritium concentration decay could be described by four exponential processes. 2) The biological half-life of the tritiated glycoside amounted to 4.2 d (^{3}H gitoxin 3.9 d) independently of the way of administration, and was determined from the terminal exponential decay of radioactivity in the plasma. The size of this phase amounted to less than 1% of the initial plasma level. 3) The onset of the terminal elimination phase (TEP) seems to coincide with the attainment of a constant parent glycoside/metabolites ratio as can be concluded from the PC and T/M remaining constant from the second day on. 4) Similarly, the fraction of tritium bound to plasma proteins decayed from 70% to 25% within two days after drug administration, and then remained constant. 5) During the TEP the T/M amounted to 10, 3, 1.5, 1.3, and 1.3 for liver, kidney, heart, skeletal muscle and medulla, respectively. 6) 1, 2 and 7 days following i. a., 23 and 11, 27 and 26, and 32 and 47% of the given dose had been excreted via urine and feces, respectively. Similar values were obtained after o.a of the drug. 7) Within the first 6 hours, the biliary excretion of radioactivity amounted to only 1/10 of that excreted with urine and feces during the same period.

Department of Pharmacology, University of Kiel, D 23 Kiel, Hospitalstrasse 4 - 6

136

MODULATION OF FUNCTIONAL AND METABOLIC OUABAIN ACTIONS BY SALICYLATE AND INDOMETHACIN K. Güttler, W. Klaus and B. Meyer

Previous studies on isolated guinea-pig hearts perfused at a constant rate with Tyrode's solution (K. Güttler and B. Meyer, Naunyn-Schmiedeberg's Arch.Pharmacol. 297,(Suppl.II),R 28, 1977; K. Güttler, W. Klaus and B. Meyer, J. Molec. Cell. Cardiol. 9, (Suppl), 17, 1977) have shown that Na-salicylate reduces the inotropic activity of ouabain and in addition shifts the manifestation of ouabain toxicity into a higher concentration range.
To elucidate further the mechanism of this interaction we compared the effects of indomethacin ($2.8 \times 1o^{-6}$M) with that of Na-salicylate (6 x $1o^{-3}$ M) on the ouabain (8 x $1o^{-7}$ M) actions in this system:
1. Salicylate reduces the positive inotropic action of ouabain whereas indomethacin does not.
2. Salicylate decreases the coronary resistance whereas indomethacin increases it.
3. Salicylate causes a retention of myocardial potassium whereas indomethacin has no influence on the myocardial potassium balance.
4. Both salicylate and indomethacin delay the onset of ouabain-induced arrhythmias by the same degree.
It is concluded that the Na-salicylate interaction with ouabain is mainly due to a membrane effect contrary to the influence of indomethacin which might be related to an interference of this substance with the myocardial prostaglandin synthesis.

Institute of Pharmacology, University of Cologne, Gleueler Str. 24, D - 5ooo Köln 41

137

ON THE SPECIFICITY OF BINDING OF PROSTAGLANDINS TO CORO-
NARY ARTERIES - CORRELATION TO THE BIOLOGICAL RESPONSE
U. Fricke and K. Schrör

The relationship of prostaglandin (PGE_1, PGE_2) binding and
biological response was studied on isolated bovine coronary
arteries. Tension development of helically cut strips was
measured isometrically (preload: 2 gms) in modified Tyrode
solution ($37^\circ C$, pH 7.4). The binding (tissue/medium ratio)
was determined simultaneously in strips of the same vessels
using 3H-PGE_1, 3H-PGE_2. Binding at conditions without biological response was estimated in Tris-buffer (5o mM, pH
7.4). The binding and biological activity of 14C-linoleic
acid (LA) was studied in the same manner. Cumulative application of PGE_2 (o.2 - 177 μM) was followed by a concentra-
tion-dependent increase in both tension development (max
= 0.79 $\pm$ o.13 g, ED-5o = 6 μM. n=7) and binding (max =
o.94 $\pm$ o.07, n=6). Pretreatment with indomethacin (3 μM)
did not alter biological response or binding (n=4). With
PGE_1 (o.o4 - 177 μM) there was a small relaxation followed
by a final contraction. Strips, previously contracted by
PGE_2 (2o μM) responded only with relaxation (max = o.46 $\pm$
o.o6 g, ED-5o = 4 μM. n=7). This was parallelled by an increase in binding (max = 1.45 $\pm$ o.06, n=6), which was significantly higher than in nonpretreated strips (max = 1.15
$\pm$ o.o3, n=6). Binding of PGE_1 and PGE_2 in Tris-buffer gave
similar curves shifted, however, to lower values (o.8o $\pm$
o.05, n=6, o.97 $\pm$ o.07, n=6). With LA (o.2 - 221 μM) there
was neither biological response nor difference in binding
between Tris and Tyrode solutions (max = 13.31 $\pm$ o.98,
n=6; max = 13.34 $\pm$ 1.02, n=6). Plotting the biological response in dependence on the tissue binding resulted in a
linear correlation over a wide concentration range (o.4-
4o μM) for both prostaglandins. This investigation of
binding close to physiological situations provides evidence for prostaglandin binding sites mediating their coronary vasomotory response. (Supported by the Deutsche
Forschungsgemeinschaft: Schr 194/2)

Pharmakologisches Institut der Universität zu Köln,
Gleueler Str. 24, D-5ooo Köln 41

138

THE INFLUENCE OF PGE_2 ON LOCAL MYOCARDIAL PER-
FUSION - A COMPARISON WITH ADENOSINE
R. Rösen and H.J. Link

Local myocardial perfusion was studied on isolated guinea pig hearts using the fluorescence
indicator technique. Wash in and wash out kinetics of fluoresceinisothiocarbamyl-dextran 3ooo
(FITC-dextran 3) as well as steady state fluorescence were continuously measured at the left
ventricular surface using a microscope fluori-
meter and correlated to the coronary flow. The
analysis of the kinetic data revealed a strong
correlation of the halftimes ($t_{1/2}$) to the coronary flow in the range of 5 - 14 ml/min. Equi-
effective concentrations of PGE_2 (1.42×10^{-8}M)
and adenosine (1×10^{-7}M) on coronary flow (increase from 7.5 to 13.5 ml/min) show an identical decrease in $t_{1/2}$ ($7o \pm$ 2% n=7, $67 \pm$ 2% n=12
of the control)indicating no difference in the
rate of fluorescence indicator exchange. In contrast PGE_2 and adenosine differed in their action
on the steady state fluorescence (F_{max}). Adenosine caused a concentration dependent increase
in F_{max} which was well correlated to the increase
in coronary flow (b_{xy}=o.75 r=o.88o, n=24). PGE_2
did not change F_{max} significantly neither in
cumulative concentration response curves nor in
single concentration experiments. These results
provide evidence for a different site of action
of adenosine and PGE_2: Adenosine increases the
perfusion volume at the ventricular surface,
whereas PGE_2 does not.
Department of Pharmacology, University of Köln,
D 5ooo Köln, Gleueler Str. 24

139

CORONARY DILATORY ACTION OF ADENOSINE ANALOGUES
IN THE ANAESTHETIZED AND AWAKE DOG. G.Raberger
J.P.Binder

The coronary dilatory action of 23 adenosine
analogues was investigated after i.v. administration in anaesthetized dogs. Substitution in
5'position with COOH and esterification or ami-
dation led to very effective compounds. The 5'
ethylcarboxamide was approximately 2oooo times
more active than adenosine,mainly because of a
marked prolongation of the action. Additional
substitution in positions 2' and 3' with NO_2,
O-methoxy-methyliden or O-methoxy-ethyliden resulted in a delayed onset and prolonged duration
of action. Since higher doses of the 2'3'5'substituted analogues were needed in comparison to
the only 5' substituted analogue,a metabolic
degradation to the 5' analogue must be assumed
for the 2'3'5' substituted analogues.
In the awake dog 2'3'-O-methoxy-ethyliden-adeno-
sine-5'ethylcarboxamide (744-98) led to marked
dose dependant increases in coronary blood flow.
A slight increase in renal blood flow was also
observed.In the standing position high doses of
744-98 revealed an adenosine-like negative chronotropic action and marked hypotension. Metabolic effects were observed with higher coronary
active doses only. The increase in arterial glucose and decrease in free fatty acid levels are
considered to be caused by glucagon-releasing
and adenosine-like actions of 744-98. The haemodynamic and metabolic actions were observed
after i.v. and oral administration, showing a
ratio of approximately 3:1 in favour of the
parenteral route.

Pharmakologisches Institut der Univ. Wien,
A 1o9o Wien, Währingerstr. 13a

140

GLUCAGON-RELEASE INDUCED BY VASOACTIVE ADENO-
SINE DERIVATIVES IN THE CONSCIOUS DOG
W. Schütz and B. Stanek

Adenosine-5'-ethylcarboxamide (744-96) and adenosine analogues additionally substituted at
the 2'- and 3'-position with an o-methoxy-
-ethylidene- (744-98) or a di-o-nitro-group
(744-99) were shown to be characterized by pronounced coronary dilatory and vasodepressor activity (Raberger et al., Arch.Int.Pharmacodyn.,
in press). The also observed metabolic effects
of these compounds were further investigated in
the present study carried out on conscious dogs
especially with regard to glucagon-releasing
activity. Heart rate and blood pressure were
measured simultaneously. Each adenosin derivative, administered iv. at a dosage of 10 μg/kg,
induced an increase in plasma glucose and a decrease in plasma FFA concentration; concomi-
tantly, plasma glucagon levels rose 2-3-fold.
Changes in plasma insulin concentration were
relatively small and of no statistical significance. With regard to metabolic and haemodynamic effects, 744-96 was the most effective compound. The glucagon-releasing activity of the
three adenosine derivatives parallels their respective vasodepressor effects. After premedi-
cation with the adenosine-antagonistic drug
aminophylline (10 mg/kg iv.) both, the vasodepressor as well as the glucagon response induced by 744-96 were markedly diminished and
plasma glucose and FFA levels remained nearly
unaltered. These results point to the presence
of identical adenosine receptors in mediating
vasodilation and glucagon secretion.

Pharmakologisches Institut der Universität,
Währinger Str. 13a, A-1090 Wien

141

QSAR-STUDIES IN THE INOTROPIC ACTION OF NIFEDI-PINE-DERIVATIVES. R.Rodenkirchen, E.Möller[+], R. Mannhold, F.Bossert[+], and H.Meyer[+]

Among the so-called calcium-antagonists one of the most potent and commonly used compounds is nifedipine. Based on an analysis of the specific inotropic action of nifedipine exerted in cat papillary muscles we have investigated the physicochemical and steric requirements for this action. The quantitative structure-activity relationships (QSAR-studies) were realized by means of a Hansch analysis:Substituent constants, describing electronic, hydrophobic and steric properties of the nifedipine-derivatives were correlated with their biological activity (ED_{50}-value for the negative inotropic effect). For a group of ortho-substituted nifedipine-derivatives significant correlations were obtained mainly with steric parameters (E_s, B_1). The following example shows the regression analysis and the statistical data obtained with the new steric Verloop-parameter B_1:

$$\log 1/ED_{50} = 5.06 + 0,8 \ (\pm 0.15) \cdot B_1$$

n=8, r=0.91, T=5.28, F=27.88, P=0.0019
In this case an increasing activity depends on an increasing size of the substituents. For a group of congeneric esters significant correlations were obtained with lipophilic and/or steric parameters (π, R_M', E_s, V_W). Now a decreasing activity depends on an increasing lipophilicity and/or size of the substituents. Here an example of the regression analysis with the lipophilic parameter R_M':

$$\log 1/ED_{50} = 6.46 - 1.65 \ (\pm 0.29) \cdot R_M'$$

n=5, r=0.96, T=-5.76, F=33.2, P=0.0104

Institut für Klinische Physiologie, Universität Düsseldorf
+Chem.wiss.Lab.Pharma, BAYER AG, Wuppertal

142

INFLUENCE OF HEXOBENDINE ON THE EFFLUX OF (^{14}C)-PURINE NUCLEOSIDES FROM ISOLATED PERFUSED GUINEA-PIG HEART   H. Wiener, W.G. Schützenberger, E. Tuisl, and N. Kolassa

Isolated guinea-pig hearts were perfused according to the Langendorff technique at constant flow with a non-recirculating modified Krebs-Henseleit solution (J.Schrader et al., Pflügers Arch. 367,129, 1976) containing 10^{-6} M of the deaminase inhibitor erythro-9-(2-hydroxy-3-nonyl)adenine. Following a labelling period (20 min, 10^{-6} M (8-^{14}C)adenosine) perfusion was continued with an adenosine-free medium. After 20 min the ^{14}C-concentration in the perfusate amounted to about 1% of the ^{14}C-concentration administered during the labelling period and its further decline proceeded very slowly. At this point hexobendine (concentration range 10^{-8}-6×10^{-6} M) was added to the perfusion medium during a 20-min period and it elicited a transient increase in ^{14}C-efflux with a maximum (about 2-fold elevation) at 0.5 - 1.0$\times10^{-6}$ M hexobendine. About 70% of the ^{14}C-label in the perfusate were identified as (^{14}C)inosine and less than 10% as (^{14}C)-adenosine by chromatographic analysis; this distribution of ^{14}C among the nucleosides was not significantly altered by hexobendine.
The results suggest that hexobendine inhibits preferentially re-uptake of purine nucleosides at the beginning of drug administration, when a higher concentration exists in the extracellular space as compared to the intracellular. Later on, the increase in purine nucleoside efflux disappears, when the hexobendine concentrations outside and inside the cells approach equilibrium thus inhibiting release and re-uptake of purine nucleosides to a similar extent.

Pharmakologisches Institut, Universität Wien, A-1090 Wien, Währingerstr. 13a.

143

Behaviour of left ventricular dimensions in anaesthetized dogs under the influence of antianginal compounds
V.B. Fiedler and J. Scholtholt

In anaesthetized dogs left ventricular outer dimensions were measured (LVOD). Additionally blood pressure (BP), heart rate (HR), left ventricular systolic (LVP) as well as enddiastolic pressure (LVEDP), dp/dt, pulmonary artery pressure (PAP), right atrial pressure (RAP) and cardiac output (CO) were registrated. Influence of various antianginal drugs on these parameters were investigated: nitroglycerin (NG), molsidomin (M), dipyridamole (D), hexobendine (H), verapamil (V), perhexilene (P), carbocromen (C), oxyfedrine (O), the ß-blocking drug propranolol (PR), and the alpha-blocking compound phentolamine (PH). LVOD were attenuated by NG (briefly) and M (long-lasting). These effects were not antagonized either by alpha- or by ß-blockade. V depressed left ventricular dp/dt and increased LVOD. O - as a ß-stimulating drug - increased ventricular performance and lowered LVOD, but these effects could be blocked by PR.
D, H, PH, and P had no influences on LVOD. C showed a tendency to diminution of LVOD. PR increased LVOD. These result suggest, that measurement of LVOD can be a useful screening model for detecting antianginal compounds, which act mainly upon the capacitance vessels. We believe that reduction in LVOD in combination with reduction of PAP and LVEDP - or RAP - referes to a "venouspooling" effect of the screened compounds which means: antianginal action. The condition is, that these effects cannot be blocked by alpha- or by ß-blockade.

Dept. Biol. Med. Res. Cassella Farbwerke Mainkur AG, 6000 Frankfurt (Main) 61, Hanauer Landstr. 526, FRG

144

ACTIVATION MECHANISMS IN SMOOTH MUSCLE OF HUMAN CORONARY ARTERIES AND THEIR SELECTIVE INHIBITION
K. Golenhofen

Tension development was recorded in 24 spiral strips of coronary arteries from 5 human hearts (excision 3-6 hours after death). The strips developed strong spontaneous activity, often with marked fluctuations of the minute-rhythm type. Nifedipine (10^{-9} to 10^{-6} mol/l) reduced the spontaneous activity and abolished the rhythmic fluctuations. The effects of nifedipine on an activation induced by high potassium concentration ($K^+= 40$ mmol/l) and on an activation induced by noradrenaline were similar to those described for canine and porcine strips (K.Golenhofen et al., Naunyn Schmiedeberg's Arch.Pharmacol. 297,Suppl.II, R 30, 1977): nifedipine partially suppressed the reactions, and the nifedipine-resistant component was suppressed by nitroprusside sodium (10^{-5} mol/l). Nitroglycerin showed little effect under conditions with strong spontaneous rhythmical activity but was very effective in suppressing the nifedipine-resistant component of the spontaneous tone. On the basis of the P-T-concept for calcium activation in smooth muscle (K.Golenhofen, in: E.Bülbring & M.F.Shuba, Raven Press, New York 1976, pp.197-202) nifedipine and nitroglycerin can be described as partial antagonists of coronary activation, nifedipine with preferential effect on the P-system and nitroglycerin with preferential effect on the T-system. Since the P-T-ratio is different in different types of activation, the effect of these drugs on pathological constrictions may differ considerably from the effects measured under conventional experimental situations.

Dept. of Physiology, University of Marburg/Lahn, Deutschhausstr.2, D-3550 Marburg/Lahn, FRG

145

PRE- AND POSTSYNAPTIC STIMULATION OF α-ADRENOCEPTORS BY B-HT 933, AN OXAZOLOAZEPINE WITH CLONIDINE-LIKE ACTIONS L. Pichler and W. Kobinger

B-HT 933 (2-amino-6-ethyl-4,5,7,8-tetrahydro-6H-oxazolo-|5,4-d|-azepin-dihydrochloride) has been shown to exert actions typical for a clonidine-like substance, inspite of a quite different chemical structure (W.Kobinger and L. Pichler,Naunyn Schmiedeberg's Arch.Pharmacol.300,39,1977). This pattern included a direct stimulation of postsynaptic α-adrenoceptors. The present investigations were concerned with possible stimulating properties of B-HT 933 at presynaptic α-adrenoceptors. Evidence for a presynaptic effect at peripheral adrenergic nerves were gained in pithed rats(pentobarbitone), electrically stimulated (50V, 2msec, 1min) at C_7-Th_1 with different frequencies. The stimulation increased the heart rate and this tachycardia was inhibited by B-HT 933 (300 µg/kg i.v.) at low (0.2Hz) but not at higher frequencies (1.6Hz). This effect of B-HT 933 was antagonized by phentolamine (5mg/kg i.v.). B-HT 933 decreased blood pressure, heart rate and spontaneous preganglionic splanchnic nerve activity in cats (chloralose) by a central nervous effect. The hypothesis was tested, whether the effect upon the splanchnic nerve is due to a presynaptically mediated decrease in central adrenergic functions. In noradrenaline depleted cats (reserpine 5mg/kg, 18 hours and α-methyl-p-tyrosine, 300mg/kg, 18 hours and 2 hours) B-HT 933 (30 µg/kg intracisternally) decreased the rate of splanchnic discharges as effectively as in controls. These results are evidence against a presynaptic effect of B-HT 933 at central adrenergic systems.

Ernst-Boehringer-Institut für Arzneimittelforschung, A-1121, Wien.

146

PHARMACODYNAMIC AND PHARMACOKINETIC ACTIONS OF MIDODRINE AND ST 1059   H.Pittner

The alpha-adrenergic stimulating agent midodrine (1-(2',5'-dimethoxyphenyl) - 2 - glycineamido - ethanol(1))is well absorbed from the gastro - intestinal tract after oral administration.Midodrine has been suggested to be the "transport form" from which the pharmacologically active main metabolite ST 1059 (1-(2',5'-dimethoxy - phenyl)-2-amino-ethanol(1))is formed by the enzymatic cleavage of glycine.
In isolated strips of the dog femoral artery , midodrine itself (10^{-8} to $3 \cdot 10^{-4}$M) was devoid of any constrictory effects,while ST 1059 led to a vasoconstriction (ED 50 = $2 \cdot 10^{-5}$ M)which in its maximum value was comparable to that of noradrenaline(ED 50 = $9.7 \cdot 10^{-7}$M).In anaesthetized rats, equimolar doses (10^{-6} to $3 \cdot 10^{-5}$ moles/kg) of midodrine (rapidly injected i.v.) and ST 1059 (slowly infused i.v.) produced identical " areas of blood pressure rise " (= blood pressure rise x duration of action) . In conscious dogs , ^{3}H - midodrine (0.1 to 1.6 mg/kg i.v.) elevated the femoral arterial blood pressure and reduced the heart rate dose-dependently. The elimination of ^{3}H- midodrine from the plasma was accompanied by the appearance of ^{3}H - ST 1059 in the plasma . Orally applied ^{3}H- midodrine (0.8 mg/kg) was completely absorbed, and ^{3}H - ST 1059 was also formed after the oral administration of ^{3}H-midodrine. The decline in heart rate was positively correlated to the plasma levels of ^{3}H - ST 1059

These experiments demonstrate that the pharmacologically active alpha-sympathomimetic agent ST 1059 is actually formed from midodrine in the organism.

CHEMIE LINZ AG,Pharmakologie, A - 4021 Linz

147

EFFECTS OF ISOPRENALINE ON THE MICROCIRCULATION IN THE CALF MUSCLES OF THE RAT STUDIED BY FLUORESCENCE VITAL MICROSCOPY. F. Vetterlein, P. Rempel, and G. Schmidt

In a previous report a reduction of the functional capillary density in skeletal muscle during an isoprenaline-induced vasodilation has been found (F. Vetterlein, G. Schmidt, N.S.Arch. Pharmacol. 297, R 31, 1977). Short lasting changes in the capillary perfusion pattern could not be proved, however, by this method, because the tissue was exposed to the dye for a relative long time (30 to 45 sec). Therefore in the present experiments a vital microscopic investigation of the microcirculation was performed. After injecting fluorescein-conjugated γ-globulin the capillaries in the surface of the gastrocnemius muscle of the rat could be observed in an incident light fluorescence microscope. Before and after the beginning of an intraarterial infusion of 0.1 µg/kg x min isoprenaline the capillary circulation in this area was recorded cinematographically during a period of 15 sec. At these times, the total blood flow in the calf muscles (in situ isolated) amounted to 6.2 $\pm$ 0.7 (control) and 11.8 $\pm$ 1.7 (isoprenaline) ml/min x 100 g ($\bar{x}$-$s_{\bar{x}}$, n = 9). In these trials 242 capillaries could be registrated, 34 of which were not perfused during the control period. 3 min after the beginning of the infusion, in all experiments a significant (p < O.01) increase in the number of capillaries with stagnant flow was found. 135 of the 242 microvessels were not perfused during this period. These data further support the view that an increase in total blood flow is not necessarily associated with an increase in the perfusion rate of all microvessels.
Institut für Pharmakologie, Universität Göttingen, Robert-Koch-Str. 40, D 3400 Göttingen

148

ACUTE CARDIOPULMONARY EFFECTS OF OXPRENOLOL OR PROPRANOLOL IN THE DOG   J. Stepanek

Anaesthetized (α-chloralose 60 mg/kg i.v. + morphine 1 mg/kg i.m.), intubated dogs showing an O_2 saturation of 90% were given 1 mg/kg oxprenolol or propranolol i.v. Each dose was given to six dogs. Haemodynamic parameters were recorded or calculated according to the standard formulae.
Injection of oxprenolol was immediately followed by an increase in heart rate (65.7%±28.4 of initial value) and cardiac output (74.7%±19.3 of initial value). The pressure in the aorta was transiently decreased. Propranolol in the same dose was followed by a decrease in heart rate (-11.1%±4.4 of initial value) and cardiac output (-11.1%±5.5 of initial value). Aortic pressure diminished slightly.
Continuous recordings of heart rate, respiration rate, minute volume and bronchial resistance by means of the Auprem apparatus (van der Heyden, Brussels) were made over a period of altogether three hours in 8 spontaneously breathing dogs anaesthetized only with α-chloralose.
Before 1 and 2 hours after the administration of 1 mg/kg oxprenolol or propranolol by inhalation, bronchial spasm was induced by inhalation of 0.05 mg/kg aerosolized acetylcholine.
Oxprenolol caused an increase in heart rate, respiration rate and minute volume. Propranolol caused an increase in respiration rate, minute volume and bronchial resistance. Acetylcholine-induced bronchial spasm (=100%) was intensified by 177.9%±88.4 (of initial value) 10 min. after the administration of propranolol and inhibited by -25.6%±11.7 (of initial value) after oxprenolol.
It seems that the intrinsic sympathomimetic activity of oxprenolol has a significant bearing on its cardiopulmonary effects in the anaesthetized dogs.
Biological Research Laboratories of the Pharmaceuticals Division of CIBA-GEIGY Limited, 4002 Basle, Switzerland.

149

^{36}CHLORIDE EFFLUX FROM NORADRENALINE-STIMULATED RABBIT AORTA INHIBITED BY SODIUM NITROPRUSSIDE AND NITROGLYCERINE.   V.A.W. Kreye, I.Schleich

Sodium nitroprusside (NP) hyperpolarizes vascular smooth muscle. Therefore we studied its effect on Na^+, K^+, and Cl^- efflux in rabbit aortae stimulated by 10^{-7}M noradrenaline (NA). Nitroglycerine (GTN) was also included in the study.-Both drugs reduced the rate of ^{36}Cl efflux from 0.072 min^{-1} with NA alone to 0.042 or 0.045 min^{-1} after addition of 10^{-5}M NP or GTN respectively, whereas relaxation induced by Ca^{++} withdrawal had no effect on Cl efflux. This suggests that NP and GTN specifically interfere with Cl conductance. In vascular smooth muscle, the equilibrium potential E_{Cl} (-20 to -30 mV) differs considerably from the membrane potential E_m (-50 to -60 mV). Thus, a decrease in Cl conductance could result in hyperpolarization of the cells, and thereby explain the vasodilator action of NP and GTN.- No effect of the drugs on ^{24}Na efflux could be observed, but a slight reduction of ^{42}K efflux which may have resulted from a reduced driving potential $E_m - E_K$.- In contrast to vascular smooth muscle, rat deferent ducts are not relaxed by NP or GTN. In this tissue, NA does not increase and NP or GTN do not decrease Cl efflux.- In contraction studies with K^+-stimulated rat aortae, replacement of Cl^- ions in the organbath solution by isethionate ions abolished the relaxant effect of NP and organic nitrates.- These findings suggest that in vascular smooth muscle Cl^- ions may be involved in the regulation of contractile tone, and that Cl conductance may be a target for the actions of drugs. (Supported by DFG within SFB 90)

IInd Physiological Institute, University of Heidelberg, D-6900 Heidelberg, Im Neuenheimer Feld 326

150

CENTRAL CARDIOVASCULAR EFFECTS OF cGMP
A. Walland, and P. Schuhmacher

Cholinergic drugs are known to increase intracellular levels of cGMP in brain and other tissues and to cause hypotension when administered into the CNS. Therefore, it was tested, whether intracerebroventricular (i.c.v.) injection of cGMP affects blood pressure and heart rate.

I.c.v.-injection of cGMP (125, 250 and 500 mcg/kg) into anaesthetized (80 mg/kg chloralose i.v.) cats caused hypotension and bradycardia which increased with the dose but showed tachyphylaxis. This effect was due to central sympathetic inhibition because blood pressure was not changed significantly by 500 mcg/kg cGMP i.c.v. in cats with spinal axotomy between C_1 and C_2. However, in these experiments vagal reflex bradycardia elicited by 0.1 mcg/kg angiotensin i.v. was augmented by cGMP. Similarly vagal reflex bradycardia in response to electrical stimulation of both carotid sinus nerves in axotomized cats was facilitated by 500 mcg/kg cGMP i.c.v. In contrast, vagal retardation of the heart in axotomized cats in response to electrical stimulation of one depressor nerve or in response to intracardiac injection of 20 mcg veratridine was inhibited by 500 mcg/kg cGMP i.c.v.
The experiments performed demonstrate both vagal and sympathetic effects of exogenous cGMP in the brain and favour its role as a second transmitter in cardiovascular centres.

Department of Pharmacology, C.H. Boehringer Sohn, D 6507 Ingelheim.

151

BLOOD-PRESSURE, PULSE-RATE AND GROWTH OF RATS DURING AN EIGHT MONTHS LOAD WITH INCREASING AMOUNTS OF CADMIUM IN DRINKING-WATER H.Fingerle

Groups of each 10 male and female Sprague-Dawley rats (initial body-weight 150-200 g) were treated with increasing concentrations of Cd (as chloride) in drinking water: 0; 5; 12.6 and 31.6 ppm. According to H.A. SCHROEDER, 1973 (Essays in Toxicol., 4, 107-199) two groups (10 male, 10 female animals) received in addition to 5 ppm Cd : 5 ppm Cu; 50 ppm Zn; 10 ppm Mn; 5 ppm Cr; 1 ppm Co and 1 ppm Mo.

Blood-pressure and pulse-rate were measured indirectly 22 times during the test period; in contrast to SCHROEDER the animals were not subjected to any anesthesia. The consumption of water and food was determined daily resp. all two days, and body-weight was recorded once a week.

Up to now, i.e., after eight months, any of the parameters was influenced significantly by Cd except drinking-water.
In additional experiments it was shown that the consumption of water is reduced by Cd in a dose dependent manner (r = 0.98 for males; r = 0.97 for males), a 50 % reduction occurs at 40 ppm Cd When saccharine (1.1 g/l) was added to the water increased amounts were taken up in the presence of Cd concentrations up to 30 ppm. These data suggest that Cd has a bad, perhaps bitter, taste for rats.

In man aqueous solutions of 30 ppm Cd are tasteless

Dep. of Nutrition, Pharmacology and Toxicology, University of Hohenheim, D-7000 Stuttgart 70, Fruwirthstrasse 14

152

ON THE RESETTING OF BARORECEPTORS. Hermann Bader.

Baroreceptors are able to reset to different blood pressure levels. This resetting is seen with local drug application to the baroreceptor area, sympathetic stimulation of the cervical ganglia, renal hypertension or primary hypertension. Based on the fact that the baroreceptors depend on the stress within the vessel wall, three different mechanisms are considered for their resetting:
1. Change of direction of baroreceptors within the vessel wall due to smooth muscle activity. Since the stress within a blood vessel is in longitudinal direction half of that in tangential direction, a change of the baroreceptors from tangential to longitudinal direction would lower their firingrate at a given blood pressure.
2. Change of the ratio of radius to wall thickness due to change of thickness of the vessel wall. Since the stress within the vessel wall depends directly on the ratio of radius to wall-thickness, any change of this ratio at a given pressure would also change the firingrate of the baroreceptors. 3. Adaptation of baroreceptors to different stress levels. Since the stress of the blood vessels decreases at a given pressure with age, the baroreceptors have to adapt to the decreasing stress in order to maintain a constant bloodpressure. A failure in adaptation would increase the firingrate of the baroreceptors with age and lead to hypertension.

Abteilung Pharmakologie und Toxikologie Universität Ulm, Oberer Eselsberg, 79 Ulm

153

SYMPATHETIC VASCULAR TONE IN SPONTANEOUSLY HYPERTENSIVE RATS
W. Rascher, A. Schömig, J.B. Lüth, M. Schmidt

Increased activity of the sympathetic nervous system may be involved in the pathogenesis of genetic hypertension of rats. In order to assess the significance of the peripheral sympathetic activity sympathetic vascular tone was studied in stroke prone spontaneously hypertensive rats (spSHR) and Wistar-Kyoto control rats (WKR) by measuring:
1) Plasma concentrations of catecholamines (CA)
2) Reactivity of the isolated perfused hindlimb vasculature to noradrenaline (NA).
CA were determined by a radioenzymatic method (M. DaPrada, G. Zürcher Life Sci. 19,1161-1174, 1976). Blood samples for the determination of CA were obtained from incision of the tail under thiobarbiturate anaethesia or from chronic femoral artery catheter in the undisturbed animal.
In 5 weeks, 12 weeks, and 28 weeks old animals NA levels are significantly higher in spSHR than in WKR. No differences were found for plasma concentrations of adrenaline and dopamine.
In 5 weeks old rats the vascular bed of the isolated perfused hindlimbs of spSHR was more sensitive to NA than that of WKR. The dose-response curve was shifted to the left and the maximum response was increased. The same enhanced responsiveness was seen in young spSHR in which the development of blood pressure increase had been delayed by dietary sodium restriction.
It is concluded that in the pathogenesis of spontaneous hypertension of rats an enhanced sympathetic vascular tone is of significance.

Department of Pharmacology and Internal Medicine III (Cardiology), University of Heidelberg
Im Neuenheimer Feld 366 D-6900 Heidelberg

154

DIFFERENCES IN CIRCADIAN RHYTHM OF BLOOD PRESSURE IN NORMOTENSIVE AND HYPERTENSIVE RATS
E.v.Möllendorff, C.Spillner, W. Bartsch and K. Dietmann

The rat is frequently used for the testing of substances acting on the blood pressure. However, no information about the spontaneous oscillation of the blood pressure of rats over a 24-hour-period has been available until now. By continuous recording of the blood pressure the circadian rhythm was evaluated in normotensive, mineralocorticoid-hypertensive and spontaneously hypertensive rats (ten of each). The implantation of the catheter into the femoral artery was carried out at least 2 weeks before the recording. For the evaluation, values of mean blood pressure were determined for every 5 minutes and averaged over 15 minutes.
The data show a circadian rhythm in all the 3 groups. In normotensive and mineralocorticoid-hypertensive rats the blood pressure level is higher during the active night hours than in the daytime. The pressure in the spontaneously hypertensive rats behaves in the converse manner. The respective minimum and maximum mean pressures were:
115 and 125 mm Hg in normotensive rats
145 and 155 mm Hg in mineralocorticoid-hypertensive rats
155 and 175 mm Hg in spontaneously hypertensive rats.
The differences in circadian behaviour may be explained by a varying sensitivity to exogeneous influences. In blood pressure studies in rats lasting some hours this circadian rhythm should be taken into account.

Pharmakologische Laboratorien, Boehringer Mannheim GmbH, D 6800 Mannheim 31, Postfach 310120

155

CENTRAL SEROTONIN MECHANISMS AND CARDIOVASCULAR CONTROL IN THE RAT   J.F. Smits

The participation of 5-hydroxytryptamine (5-HT, serotonin) in central cardiovascular control is less well investigated than that of noradrenaline. 5-HT (0.001-10 µg) was injected stereotaxically into the diencephalon of pentobarbital (50 mg/kg, i.p.) anaesthetized male Wistar rats. Blood pressure was recorded from the right carotid artery and heart rate was determined from the blood pressure recording. Only when injected specifically into the anterior hypothalamic-preoptic region (AH/PO) 5-HT caused an increase in arterial blood pressure, a significant increase of $^+8 \pm 2$ mm Hg already occurring after a dose of 0.01 µg 5-HT (N=6). Heart rate was not affected at any of the doses injected. Injections outside of the AH/PO region did not influence blood pressure or heart rate.
Since the majority of CNS 5-HT cell bodies in the rat are located in the dorsal and median raphe nuclei, these nuclei were stimulated electrically using stereotaxically implanted electrodes. Stimulation of each of the raphe nuclei caused an increase in blood pressure without affecting heart rate. The size of the increase in blood pressure depended upon the stimulus intensity. 5 Sec trains of 0.3 msec, 300 µA stimuli given at a frequency of 50 Hz caused an increase of $^+22 \pm 3$ mm Hg (N=22) after median raphe stimulation, whereas the same parameters applied to the dorsal raphe increased blood pressure by $^+23 \pm 5$ mm Hg (N=12). These parameters were ineffective when applied to regions outside of the raphe nuclei.
Pretreating rats with the 5-HT depletor para-chlorophenylalanine (100 mg/kg daily for 3 days, i.p.) significantly antagonized the increases in blood pressure obtained after electrical stimulation of the median raphe nucleus, but not those seen after dorsal raphe stimulation.
These data indicate a pressor role for CNS raphe-hypothalamic 5-HT neurones.

Department of Pharmacology, Rijksuniversiteit Limburg, Postbus 616, Maastricht, The Netherlands.

156

THE CENTRAL EFFECT OF PHYSOSTIGMINE ON BLOOD PRESSURE AND HEART RATE; POSSIBLE CHOLINERG ASPECTS OF BLOOD PRESSURE REGULATION
D. de Wildt and A.J. Porsius

In recent years it has been established that central adrenergic mechanisms are involved in the regulation of blood pressure. However, less information is available concerning the central effects of cholinergic drugs on haemodynamics. In the few studies published the various authors have obtained controversial results concerning the effects of centrally administered cholinergic drugs on blood pressure.
This problem was studied in a systematic manner, using the lipophilic cholinesterase inhibitor physostigmine. The central actions of this drug on blood pressure and cardiac frequency were investigated by infusing very low doses in the left vertebral artery of the anaesthetized cat. The low doses gave rise to a dose dependent decrease in blood pressure. A dose as low as 2.7 µg/kg reduced blood pressure by about 35%. High doses caused bradycardia. Occlusion of the right vertebral artery shifted the dose-response curve to the left. It seems likely that the hypotension was due to stimulation of muscarinic receptors in the pontomedullary region, since pretreatment with dexetimide administered via the vertebral artery strongly reduced the effect. Bilateral cervical vagotomy did not change the hypotensive action of physostigmine. This observation might suggest a reduction of sympathetic outflow as the possible cause of the depressor effect. After intravenous administration only doses higher than 28 µg/kg evoked hypotension, which could not be blocked by intravenously administered N-methyl-atropine. However, centrally infused dexetimide considerably antagonized this effect indicating that the hypotension was brought about by a central action and not induced peripherally. Porsius et al. (in press) suggested a transmitter role for ACh in the central haemodynamic control. This presumption is supported by the present experimental data obtained with physostigmine.

Department of Pharmacy, Division of Pharmacotherapy, University of Amsterdam,
Plantage Muidergracht 24, Amsterdam, The Netherlands.

157

CARDIOVASCULAR ACTIONS AND PHARMACOKINETICS OF PROPRANOLOL IN THE SPONTANEOUSLY HYPERTENSIVE RAT H. Struyker-Boudier

Variable cardiovascular effects have been reported after the administration of propranolol in animals. We have injected d,l-propranolol (P) subcutaneously (s.c. 0.04-5 mg/kg) or intracerebroventricularly (i.vt. 0.04 and 0.2 mg/kg) into conscious SHR. Mean arterial blood pressure (MAP) and heart rate (HR) were recorded continuously. The degree of β receptor blockade was determined from isoprenaline (ISO) induced changes in MAP and HR 1 hour before and $\frac{1}{2}$, $1\frac{1}{2}$, 3 and 20 hrs. after P injection. I.vt. injection of P caused an immediate increase in MAP of 15 ± 5 (0.04 mg/kg, N=6) and 21 ± 5 (0.2 mg/kg, N=6) mm Hg. After 0.2 mg/kg MAP was significantly lower than saline control levels 6-20 hrs. after the P injection with a maximum fall of 48 ± 15 mm Hg at 12 hrs. S.c. injection of P only increased MAP significantly after 5 mg/kg (12 ± 2 mm Hg, N=8). 0.2 Mg/kg or higher doses caused a decrease of MAP below control level at 4-20 hrs. after the injection, with a maximum fall of 38 ± 12 (0.2 mg/kg, N=6) or 58 ± 17 mm Hg (5 mg/kg, N=8). Both after i.vt. and s.c. injection HR dropped immediately. The degree of bradycardia did not differ for the routes of administration. Maximum bradycardia was observed after 10-30 min., the effect lasting 1-2 hrs. ISO-induced hypotension and tachycardia were significantly antagonized by 0.2 mg/kg P i.vt. or 0.2-5 mg/kg P s.c. The degree of antagonism was maximal at $\frac{1}{2}$ hr. and lasted $1\frac{1}{2}$-3 hrs.   In order to study the pharmacokinetic behavior of P in SHR, 1 mg/kg P was injected s.c. A plasma peak concentration of 0.38 ± 0.03 µg/ml (N=10) was obtained after 5 min. Concentration then rapidly declined with $t\frac{1}{2}\alpha$ and $t\frac{1}{2}\beta$ of 27 and 82 min. In heart, brain and lung maximal P conc. was observed between 5 and 30 min. Total P metabolite conc. in plasma and tissues increased rapidly during 15-30 min. after injection and remained high for prolonged periods. These data indicate that P-induced β-receptor blockade and bradycardia - in contrast to hypotension - follow plasma and heart kinetic profile of P.

Department of Pharmacology, Rijksuniversiteit Limburg, Postbus 616, Maastricht, The Netherlands.

158

LONG TERM STUDY OF THE ANTIHYPERTENSIVE EFFECT OF PYROXAMIDINE (EMD 21 192) IN RENAL-HYPERTENSIVE DOGS.
E. Schorscher, H.-J. Schliep, K.-O. Mink and Th. Wolf.

Pyroxamidine (1,2,3,4,10,10a-Hexahydropyrazino(1,2-a)-indolcarboxamidinium-(2)-chlorid), a new compound inhibiting the sympathoadrenal system has shown antihypertensive activity in animal studies as well as in initial clinical trials. In four renalhypertensive mongrel-dogs with carotis loops Pyroxamidine (P.) has been dosed at 6.5 mg/kg in Gelatine-capsules once per day for 10 and 95 days. Blood pressure war measured by tonometry at the carotis-loop daily prior to the administration of P. or empty capsules for the whole duration of the study.
P. induced a continous decrease of blood pressure during the first days of treatment. After the 6th day pressure values reached a stable level of about 40 mm Hg lower than the initial values, which was maintained during the whole period of drug administration. Pulse rate showed a minor decrease by about 10 - 15 pulses/minute. Discontinuation of drug administration resulted in a increase in blood pressure, evident after 4 - 6 days. In all four dogs blood pressure reached the initial values after 20 - 22 days. Tyramine (i.v.) induced blood pressure increase was diminished but not blocked during treatment with P. as compared to the period before treatment and after recovery. Interruption of treatment with P. did not show any influence on the effect of P. after reinstating the treatment. Development of drug tolerance, impairment of cardiovascular function or noxious effects on the adrenosympathetic system have not been noticed.

Department of Pharmacology, E. Merck, D 61 Darmstadt, Frankfurter Str. 250

159

CENTRAL HYPOTENSIVE ACTIVITY AS A FUNCTION OF PERIPHERAL HYPERTENSIVE POTENCY AND LIPOPHILICITY
P.B.M.W.M. Timmermans

Recently, we could establish a linear relationship between the central hypotensive and the peripheral hypertensive activities for 13 clonidine-like imidazolidines in which the difference in accessibility to the receptive sites was accounted for quantitatively by the octanol/buffer (pH=7.4) partition coefficients (Europ.J.Pharmacol., 45, 229, 1977). This finding indicates that possibly the central and the peripheral, vascular α-adrenoceptors make identical demands upon the molecular structure of their agonists. In order to verify this conclusion similar correlation studies were performed for 16 structurally very dissimilar α-adrenoceptor agonists. The compounds studied involved structures with different bridges, hetero rings, aromatic and non-aromatic moieties. Their hypotensive activities, mediated by stimulation of central α-adrenoceptors at medullary sites, were determined from dose-response curves after administration to pentobarbitone-anaesthetized, normotensive rats. Their hypertensive potencies, caused by excitation of peripheral, vascular α-adrenoceptors were quantified similarly in pithed rats. Apparent partition coefficients (log P') between octanol/aqueous buffer (pH=7.4) at $37°C$ were employed to describe the difference in accessibility to these receptors. For these structurally dissimilar α-adrenoceptor-stimulating agents again a most significant relationship was found between the central hypotensive activity and a linear combination of peripheral hypertensive potency and lipophilicity (log P'). It appears that upon including very lipophilic substances a parabolic description in log P' is necessary. The results indicate a resemblance among the central α-adrenoceptors at medullary sites and those located in the periphery at the vascular wall, at least towards these agonists.

Department of Pharmacy, Division of Pharmacotherapy, University of Amsterdam, Plantage Muidergracht 24, Amsterdam, The Netherlands.

160

THE ANTAGONISM OF THE ANTIHYPERTENSIVE ACTION OF CLONIDINE BY BETA-SYMPATICOLYTIC AGENTS IN THE SH-RAT
R. Sloos

The effects of the combination of clonidine and beta-sympaticolytic agents on blood-pressure have not yet been investigated thoroughly. In clinical literature an antagonism between clonidine and sotalol has been reported by Saarimaa (Brit.Med.J. 1976, 2, 810). We investigated the effects of clonidine and various beta-sympaticolytic agents on blood pressure and cardiac frequency during chronic treatment of spontaneously hypertensive rats. Systolic blood pressure and heart rate were measured in conscious rats, using the tail-cuff method. SH-rats were given clonidine 100 µg/kg once daily via an intragastric tube during 2 weeks, after which the beta-sympaticolytic agents were added to the regimen, using the same route of administration. Blood pressure and cardiac frequency were measured on several days about 2 hours after administration of the drugs. Results: (systolic blood pressure $\pm$ SEM): I. control group 230 ± 4.6 mm Hg (n=6), clonidine 190 ± 4.9, (n=7), clonidine $\pm$ propanolol 10 mg/kg 209 ± 5.7 (n=8). II. control group 223 ± 3.7 (n=10), clonidine 204 ± 3.0 (n=9), clonidine + sotalol 30 mg/kg 233 ± 3.0 (n=9). III. control group 219 ± 5.1 (n=7), clonidine 209 ± 3.6 (n=8), clonidine + atenolol 10 mg/kg 198 ± 5.4 (n=8). Conclusions: addition of propanolol or sotalol after chronic pretreatment with clonidine results in a significant increase of systolic blood pressure (p<0.01). In the case of sotalol the effect was even stronger than in the control group (p<0.05). Addition of the beta-1 selective agent atenolol results in a slight decrease of systolic BP, which is, however, statistically not significant (p = $\pm$ 0.10). These results suggest an antagonism at the level of peripheral beta-2 receptors.

Department of Pharmacy, Division of Pharmacotherapy, University of Amsterdam, Plantage Muidergracht 24, Amsterdam, The Netherlands.

161

INCREASED CENTRAL HYPOTENSIVE AND BRADYCARDIC ACTIVITY OF CLONIDINE AFTER MODIFICATION OF THE VERTEBRAL ARTERY TECHNIQUE

M.A. el Sherbini-Schepers and P.A. van Zwieten

A centrally mediated hypotensive and bradycardic effect of clonidine has been demonstrated upon infusion of this drug into the left vertebral artery (V.A.) of anaesthetized cats (R.W. Sattler and P.A. van Zwieten, Europ.J.Pharmacol. 2, 9, 1967). According to Reneman et al. (Cardiovasc.Res. 8, 65, 1974), infusion of radio-labelled microspheres into the left V.A. of the cat results in an accumulation of microspheres at the left side of the brain stem and cerebellum. This monolateral distribution can be explained by the laminar flow in the basilar artery. This flow pattern can be disturbed by occlusion of the opposite V.A. (D.A. Mc Donald and J.M. Potter, J.Physiol. 114, 356, 1951). We have studied the effect of centrally injected clonidine on mean arterial pressure (MAP) and heart rate (HR) and also the distribution of the 14-C-labelled compound within the ponto-medullary (PM)-area in animals where the opposite (right) V.A. had been ligated.

After ligation of this artery the maximal decrease in MAP and HR is significantly enhanced: 58 and 18% respectively, versus 35 and 5% upon infusion into an animal with an intact right V.A. The distribution studies have demonstrated a high concentration of clonidine in the PM-area 2 min. after its application. In both models the quantity of clonidine, recovered from the total brain is about 25% of the injected dose, half of this amount is found in the PM-area. After ligation of the right V.A. the left to right transfer of the drug is increased. The ratio of the concentrations in the left and the right side of the PM-area is decreased from 16 in the normal to 2.5 in the modified V.A. model. In conclusion, ligation of the right V.A. considerably increases the sensitivity towards clonidine injected into the left V.A. and seems to be an improvement of the classical V.A.-model.

Department of Pharmacy, Division of Pharmacotherapy, University of Amsterdam, Plantage Muidergracht 24, Amsterdam, The Netherlands.

162

CLONIDINE WITHDRAWAL IN THE RAT

G. Prop

After withdrawal of the antihypertensive drug clonidine (Catapresan R) a so called "rebound" phenomenon has been described to occur. (Hökfelt, Hedeland and Dymling, Eur.J. Pharmacol. 10, 89 (1970). Blood pressure and or cardiac frequency rose to levels exceeding those before treatment. Our aim has been to mimic this phenomenon in an animal model and to study its mechanism. So far, our studies have been carried out in the rat. Blood pressure and frequency recordings were performed with conscious animals, either via a cannulated iliac artery or by means of the tail cuff method. After the abrupt cessation of a daily treatment of 100 μg clonidine per kg, intraperitoneally injected for two or three weeks we could show a significant difference in blood pressure between clonidine-treated normotensive rats and controls, which appeared 25 hours after the last injection. Oral treatment via the drinking water resulted in a difference between controls and treated animals after withdrawal only at a dosage of 50 μg kg day. At higher clonidine doses we observed high pressures and frequencies after the termination of the treatment, but also during the treatment high values were sometimes seen as well. In spontaneous hypertensive rats a rebound phenomenon could not be demonstrated. The chronic treatment with clonidine, an agent which lowers peripheral sympathetic activity, did not result in a change of sensitivity of the cardiovascular system towards noradrenaline, whilst for adrenaline a slight fall in sensitivity was established. The activity of the enzyme tyrosine hydroxylase was not altered in the pontomedullary region of the brain after the withdrawal of the drug. In the adrenals the activity of this enzyme proved reduced. Accordingly, whatever the cause of the withdrawal phenomenon in the rat may be it seems improbable that a change in sensitivity for catecholamines is responsible for it. If there occur changes in the catecholamine metabolism in the brain at all, the tyrosine hydroxylase activity is probably not a suitable parameter to measure them. Department of Pharmacy, Division of Pharmacotherapy, University of Amsterdam, Plantage Muidergracht 24, Amsterdam, The Netherlands.

163

INHIBITION OF THE RENIN-ANGIOTENSIN-SYSTEM (RAS) IN RATS WITH HEREDITARY HYPOTHALAMIC DIABETES INSIPIDUS (DI)

J.F.E. Mann, R. Dietz, B. Korte and F. Gross

Experiments were carried out in DI rats in order to answer the following questions: 1) Does furosemide have an antidiuretic action in DI rats? 2) Is the antidiuretic action due to a stimulation of the RAS? I) DI rats (n=10) were placed in metabolic cages. Saline (5 ml/kg) and furosemide (50 mg/kg) were injected intraperitoneally (i.p.). Cumulative urine volume (UV)(2 and 6 h after treatment) and urinary sodium excretion (UNa$^+$)(6 h after treatment) were measured. Furosemide elicited an increase of UV during the first 2 h (21.4 ± 0.7 vs 14.5 ± 1.2 ml in controls) but a reduction of UV from the 2nd to the 6th h (5.1 ± 1.2 vs 31.2 ± 2.8ml). Total UV also decreased for the whole 6 h period in the furosemide treated rats (26.5 ± 1.2 vs 45.7 ± 3.8 ml). UNa$^+$ was enhanced to 1336 ± 72 vs 358 ± 52 μEq by furosemide treatment. II) A converting enzyme inhibitor (SQ 14225, 2.5 mg/kg) was given orally in DI rats (n=9) in order to block the conversion of angiotensin I to angiotensin II. The experimental design was as described in I). SQ 14225 elicited an increase of UV 2 h (16.6 ± 2.5 vs 8.3 ± 1.5 ml) and 6 h (44.9 ± 2.6 vs 28.8 ± 1.6 ml) after treatment. III) Furosemide treatment (50 mg/kg) was combined with administration of SQ 14225 (2.5 mg/kg) in DI rats (n=9)using the experimental design as in I) and II). This resulted in an increase of UV as compared with DI rats receiving furosemide only (2 h after treatment: 27.2 ± 1.6 vs 17.9 ± 1.1 ml; 6 h: 31.1 ± 1.2 vs 19.8 ± 1.4 ml). However, the reduction of UV following furosemide from the 2nd to the 6th h was not altered by SQ 14225 (2 ± 0.9 vs 3.9 ± 0.9 ml). The results show that in DI rats furosemide elicits an initial diuresis followed by an antidiuresis. The acute diuresis is aggravated by inhibition of the RAS. This inhibition, however, does not alter the antidiuresis. Our results do not support the hypothesis that the RAS mediates the antidiuretic effect of furosemide in DI rats.

Department of Pharmacology, University of Heidelberg Im Neuenheimer Feld 366, D-69 Heidelberg, FRG

164

INFLUENCE OF PROPRANOLOL ON THE CENTRAL EFFECTS OF ANGIOTENSIN.

W. Simon, A.K. Johnson, G. Wiedemann, D. Ganten.

The effects of beta-adrenergic blockade on the central effects of angiotensin II (AII) i.e. blood pressure increase and water intake were investigated.

1) Male Sprague-Dawley rats (300-350 g) received an infusion of a) solvent (n=7), b) 386 nmol (n=8) and c) 772 nmol (n=7) L-propranolol into the lateral brain ventricle (i.v.t.). The infusion rate was 2 ul/min over a period of 10 min. Arterial blood pressure (BP) was recorded continuously via a femoral artery catheter. BP increased in the propranolol-infused rats (p<0.001) but heart rate was not affected. Twenty-four h later, AII was infused at doses of 0.96, 9.6, 95.6 and 956 pmol/min. The increase of blood pressure following i.v.t. AII was reduced(p<0.05) in both groups of propranolol-treated rats.

2) Male Wistar rats (350-400g) received a) propranolol diet (95.6 μmol·kg^{-1} per day, n=12) or b) a control diet (n=12). After 16 days BP was unchanged, while the heart rate was reduced in the propranolol-treated rats (p< 0.001). BP responses following i.v.t. AII showed a significant reduction at the highest dose of AII. The drinking response to 95.6 pmol AII i.v.t. was also reduced in the propranolol-treated rats (p<0.05).

We conclude that i.v.t. AII effects are inhibited by propranolol. This suggests a participation of the adrenergic system in central AII effects on blood pressure and drinking.

Dept. of Pharmacology, University of Heidelberg, Im Neuenheimer Feld 366, D-6900 Heidelberg.

165

COMPONENTS OF THE RENIN-ANGIOTENSIN SYSTEM IN CE-
REBROSPINAL FLUID (CSF) AND IN PERIVENTRICULAR
BRAIN TISSUE. P.Schelling, G.Sponer, U.Ganten

The regulatory capacity of components of the
brain renin-angiotensin system was investigated.

1) Rats were implanted with a cannula into the
lateral brain ventricle and a catheter into the
femoral artery. They were then infused intraven-
tricularly (i.v.t.) with a 3600-fold purified human renin preparation. Arterial blood pressure
increased from 110 ± 4.5 to 138 ± 5.3 mm Hg (means$\pm$
SEM). This effect could be blocked by i.v.t. infusion of the angiotensin II (AII) antagonist Saralasin. The angiotensin I (AI) concentration in
CSF after infusion of the purified brain enzyme
increased from 0 to 147.9 ± 18.8 fmol $AI\cdot ml^{-1}$.

2) No angiotensinase activity was detectable in
CSF of rats. Incubation of AI with CSF led to a
decrease of AI concentration and generation of
AII in stechiometric relationships. This AI-con-
verting enzyme activity was 7.4 ± 0.1 ng $AII\cdot ml^{-1}\cdot$
h^{-1}. Angiotensinase activity in the subfornical
organ (1093 ± 91 ng AII degraded$\cdot$mg $protein^{-1}\cdot h^{-1}$)
and in the subcommissural organ (1094 ± 61 ng) was
found to be higher than in all other periventricular tissues studied such as organum vasculosum
lamina terminalis (660 ± 38 ng) and anterior 3rd
ventricle surrounding tissue (729 ± 29 ng).

The results show that brain renin can act on endogenous angiotensinogen in CSF to form AI which
is converted to AII by the converting enzyme present in CSF. Degradation of AII takes place in
contact with periventricular tissue and not in
CSF.

Department of Pharmacology, University of Heidelberg, Im Neuenheimer Feld 366, D-6900 Heidelberg.

166

POSTOCCLUSIVE RESPONSE OF RENAL BLOOD FLOW IN THE CAT

H. Osswald and W.S. Spielman

In contrast to the postocclusive hyperemia of brain, heart,
and skeletal muscle, the hemodynamic response of the kidney following renal artery occlusion is highly variable in
that both hyperemia and ischemia have been reported. The
present study evaluates the factors influencing the renal
response to complete renal artery occlusion (5-60 sec) in
the pentobarbital (30 mg/kg) anesthetized cat. Renal
blood flow (RBF) was measured with an electromagnetic flow
meter. Minimal postocclusive RBF is expressed as percentage decrease of preocclusion RBF. Marked postocclusive
vasoconstriction could only be demonstrated in meclofenamate (10 mg/kg) treated cats. $\Delta\%$ RBF (30 sec occlusion)
was in controls 16 ± 4 and after meclofenamate 54 ± 4
(n=10; p < .001). Chronic denervation of the kidney,
adrenergic receptor blockade (phenoxybenzamine or phentolamine), or infusion of 1-Sar-8-Ile-angiotensin II (2 µg/
min·kg) did not affect the postocclusive reduction of RBF,
indicating that the vasoconstriction was independent of
renal nerves, catecholamines and circulating angiotensin
II. Adenosine when injected into the renal artery of 5
cats caused a dose dependent transient fall of RBF. 100
nmol adenosine reduced RBF by $44\pm6\%$ whereas after meclofenamate only 1 nmol produced the same degree of vasoconstriction. Since adenosine accumulates in the kidney
several fold following renal artery occlusion (Osswald et
al., Pflügers Arch. 371:45, 1977) and the renal vasculature was 100-fold more sensitive to adenosine induced
vasoconstriction after meclofenamate treatment we suggest
that the response of the renal vasculature following renal
artery occlusion is mediated by intrarenal adenosine.
Prostaglandins, particularly in the anesthetized animal,
can mask the postocclusive vasoconstriction in the kidney.

Dept. of Pharmacology, RWTH Aachen, Melatenerstr. 213,
51 Aachen, Fed. Rep. of Germany, and Dept. of Physiology
& Biophysics, Mayo Clinic, Rochester, MN 55901 USA.

167

DISSOCIATION OF THE VASCULAR AND NATRIURETIC EFFECTS OF
DIURETIC AGENTS
J. Kraetz, L. Criscione and P.R. Hedwall

Diuretic agents of various types and chemical structures
exert a vasodilator effect which can be demonstrated as
inhibition of noradrenaline-induced vasoconstriction in
the isolated, perfused mesenteric artery preparation of
the rat. The potency of diuretic agents in this preparation: (GP 48 674 /6-methyl-5-(2-methylene-butyrylbenzo-
furane-2-carbonic acid/ > indapamide, ethacrynic acid,
bumetanide, furosemide > hydrochlorothiazide, chlorthalidone > acetazolamide) does not conform to the order of
their natriuretic potency following oral administration
in the rat: (hydrochlorothiazide, chlorthalidone, indapamide > acetazolamide > furosemide, bumetanide), and inhibition is also produced by diuretics (GP 48 674, ethacrynic acid) which do not exhibit a diuretic effect in
the rat.
The vascular effects of the diuretic agents can also be
demonstrated as inhibition of pressor responses to angio-
tensin-II and noradrenaline in the despinalized rat preparation and, less prominently, in the intact anesthetized
rat following repeated oral administration.
Since the original report of a divergence between the
vascular and diuretic effects of furosemide in man (Biagi
and Bapat: Lancet 1967/I: 849), a number of clinical pub-
lications describe a vasodilator action of various
diuretics in man, which is apparently independent of the
natriuretic activity of these agents. This dissociation
is even more prominent in the rat.

Biological Research Laboratories of the Pharmaceuticals
Division of CIBA-GEIGY Limited, 4002 Basle, Switzerland.

168

ON THE MODE OF ACTION OF DIURETICS. A STUDY BY
CONTINUOUS MICROPERFUSION OF SINGLE LOOPS OF HEN-
LE OF THE RAT KIDNEY IN VIVO   J. Greven, B.
Förster, and K. Meywald

In the intact rat, short loops of HENLE were
perfused using a technique similar to that described by CORTNEY et al. (Pflügers Arch., 287,
286-295, 1966). The perfusion fluid was a modified Ringer solution and contained 2.5 mg/ml
inulin ^{3}H and 2 mg/ml lissamine green. The drugs
studied were added to this solution. Furosemide
(10^{-7} to 10^{-3} M) decreased fluid, sodium and
chloride reabsorption in the loops. Complete inhibition of fluid and NaCl reabsorption was observed at 10^{-3} M. Perfusions with sodium or
chloride free solutions (choline chloride,
Na_2SO_4) indicated that chloride transport is
primary inhibited by this drug. Hydrochlorothiazide (10^{-5} to 10^{-3} M) also diminished the loops
reabsorptive capacity, the inhibitory effect,
however, was considerably smaller than that observed after furosemide. Furosemide, but not
hydrochlorothiazide, induced a potassium secretion into the loops at doses ranging from 10^{-5}
to 10^{-3} M. Diazoxide which chemically is closely related to hydrochlorothiazide, decreased arterial blood pressure, GFR, and urinary fluid
excretion and increased renal blood flow (electromagnetic flowmeter) after intravenous injection into rats. Microperfusion experiments revealed, that diazoxide did not stimulate fluid
and electrolyte reabsorption in the loops. It is
assumed that the antidiuretic effect of diazoxide is caused mainly by a fall of the GFR.

Department of Pharmacology, TH Aachen, D-5100
Aachen, Melatenerstr. 213.

169

Investigations on the Renal and Biliary Excretion of Furosemide and its Metabolites in Rhesus Monkeys (Macaca mulatta).
Sörgel,F.,R.Muschaweck,E.Mutschler and M.Hropot
Pharmacological properties of Furosemide(F) in Rhesus Monkeys were found to be similar to those observed in man and other animal species. Renal function parameters(GFR,endogenous Creatinine-Clearance,PAH-Clearance)were determined. A rapid and sensitive method for the simultaneous determination of F and its metabolites was developed using high performance liquid chromatography (HPTLC)analogous to that of SCHÄFER,GEISSLER, MUTSCHLER(1977). Constant plasma levels of F were maintained by infusing F at a constant infusion rate(0.01-20mg/kg/min). The Renal Clearance of F was up to 4 times higher than the actual GFR,as found with Inulin-Clearance. This supports a tubular secretion of F in the Rhesus Monkey as was previously reported for other animals. (GAYER 1964,DEETJEN,1966,CALSENDESK 1966,HROPOT and MUSCHAWECK 1976).In biliary fistulated Rhesus Monkeys it was shown that F increases bile flow. Unchanged F was present in bile at concentrations higher than in plasma. Probenecid(50mg/kg)injected as a bolus blocked the excretion of F into urine and bile. 4-Chloro-5-sulfamoylanthranilic acid(Saluamine),a possible metabolite of F,was found in bile. Conjugates of F,known from our earlier studies to form the major metabolic component,were present in plasma,urine and bile; the highest concentrations were found in bile.

HOECHST AG, D 6230 Frankfurt(M)Postfach 800320 and Pharmakologisches Institut f. Naturwissenschaftler, D 6000 Frankfurt(M) Robert-Mayer-Str. 7 - 9

170

CLINICAL STUDIES ON THE EFFECT, MODE OF ACTION AND PHARMACOKINETIC OF MUZOLIMINE.
D. Loew

Muzolimine is a saluretic from a new class of chemical substance. Like furosemide, muzolimine is initially very effective. In contrast to furosemide, however, the effect of muzolimine is prolonged. In oedema-free volunteers the threshold dose is 0.15 mg/kg.
A dose increase causes an almost linear increase in the efficacy. The pattern of action is characterised by the intensified excretion of chloride and sodium, a moderate excretion of calcium, magnesium and potassium whilst the excretion of bicarbonate remains uninfluenced. The onset of effect is rapid. The maximal effect occurs within the first two hours; the duration of effect is 6-8 hours. The average half life of muzolimine is 4 hours. The time-response curves for the excretion of sodium and urine and the drop in the concentration of muzolimine in the plasma are closely correlated. The inulin clearance is unchanged, the PAH-clearance increases in the acute saluretic phase.
Based on the free-water clearance it is assumed that the site of action is in the medullary part of the ascending limb of the Henle's loop. Muzolimine is effective, even in patients having a reduced filtration rate of 3 ml/min.

Pharma-Forschungszentrum der BAYER AG
D-5600 Wuppertal-1

171

ON THE CHARACTERIZATION OF VARIOUS EXPERIMENTAL KIDNEY DAMAGES BY CLEARANCE EXPERIMENTS ON UNANESTHETIZED RATS
G. Vogel and E. Leng

In order to investigate the extent and location of the renal lesions induced by several different agents male rats were given puromycin aminonucleoside 100 mg/kg s.c.,uranyl nitrate 2 mg/kg i.p. and mercuric chloride 1 mg/kg i.p. Twenty four hours before the renal damage reached its peak a capsule filled with inulin/PAH mixture was implanted intraperitoneally by the method of SADJAK et al. The following measurements were then carried out: urine output, GFR, absolute and fractional fluid reabsorption, PAH clearance, absolute and fractional reabsorbed/secreted amounts of urea, Na^+ and glucose. Urine protein was also determined.
Results: Aminonucleoside causes severe proteinuria, which points to a lesion predominantly at the level of the glomeruli. The protein that is excreted with the urine originates – as shown by an immunological analysis – from the plasma. The permeability of the glomerular capillaries to polyvinylpyrrolidone M.W. 110,000 is, in contrast to what one would expect, not increased.
Uranyl nitrate affects mainly the tubules. The PAH clearance falls to approximately 5% of normal, and the proportion of glucose reabsorbed is only 60% of that filtered through the glomeruli, as compared with 99% in healthy rats.
In renal damage caused by mercuric chloride both GFR and PAH clearance are reduced, though the latter is more severely affected than the former. Plasma urea rises to almost 10 times normal, while glucose reabsorption falls to half its normal value. These results indicate that mercuric chloride damages both the glomeruli and the tubules.

+) Naunyn-Schmiedeberg's Arch. Pharmakol. Suppl II Vol. 297, R 36 (1977)

Dr. Madaus u. Co., Pharmakologische Abtlg.
D - 5000 Köln 91, Ostmerheimer Str. 198

172

RELEASE OF ENDORPHINS FROM VARIOUS TISSUE EXTRACTS   W. Kromer, C. Fischer, L. Magner,and E. de la Gala

Little information is available indicating a physiological role of the endorphins. In view of a possible function of endorphins in pregnancy or birth we searched in the uterus for endorphins as well as for a factor able to stimulate the release of endorphins from the pituitary; by release of such compounds from the uterus during labour, analgesia or inhibition of intestinal motility might be achieved. Acid extracts of guinea pig uterine tissue from various stages of oestrus cycle or gestation were all found to contain about equally small amounts of endorphins as determined in opiate receptor binding assays. When the extracts were incubated at 37°C in Tris/HCl buffer (0.05 M; pH 7.4) together with peptic enzymes such as trypsin or with anterior lobe tissue from porcine pituitaries, considerable amounts of endorphins were found in the incubation medium. This might indicate the presence of a precursor molecule in the uterus extracts, from which an endorphin might have been cleaved off by the peptidases or by a pituitary enzyme. In view of these results, however, the presence of a factor in the uterus extracts able to elicit the release of endorphins from pituitary tissue cannot be excluded. Further investigations, in which anterior lobe tissue was superfused at 37°C with Krebs-Ringer solution containing uterus extracts or 50 mM potassium, also indicate the possibility that such a factor might exist in the uterus playing a role as described for releasing hormones of hypothalamic origin.

Pharmakologisches Institut der Universität München, Nußbaumstrasse 26, 8000 München 2.

173

ORGAN DISTRIBUTION AND BIOLOGICAL ACTIVITY OF 125-I-LABELLED LH-RH ANALOGUES   Sandow,J.,
W.v.Rechenberg, G.Jerzabek, W.Stoll and H.Strecker

The high biological activity of certain LH-RH analogues may be due to increased receptor binding and/or reduced enzyme stability. The organ distribution of 125-I-labelled analogues was studied to estimate the in vivo degree of receptor binding and the inactivating tissues. The following peptides were labelled with 125-I by the chloramine-T method: LH-RH(1-9)nonapeptide-ethylamide, [D-Glu^6] LH-RH(1-9)nonapeptide-ethylamide,[D-Ser(Bu^t)^6] LH-RH(1-9)nonapeptide-ethylamide and the corresponding (3-9)heptapeptide fragment. Biological activity was tested in ovariectomized, steroid-blocked rats by LH-release. Organ distribution was determined 15, 30 and 60 minutes after iv-injection of labelled peptides. After iodination, biological activity was retained to 30-50 %. The order of potency of the labelled analogues was LH-RH: LH-RH(1-9)EA:[D-Glu^6]LH-RH(1-9)EA:[D-Ser (Bu^t)^6]EA= 1:2:20:40.Pituitary accumulation of the weak analogue LH-RH(1-9)EA was only found after 15 minutes (tissue/plasma ratio 1.23), [D-Glu^6]LH-RH(1-9)EA reached a T/P ratio of 1.33 after 30 minutes and the highly active [D-Ser(Bu^t)^6] LH-RH(1-9)EA reached high pituitary accumulation even after 60 minutes (T/P ratio 2.33). The peptides were also concentrated in liver and kidney, the main inactivating organs for LH-RH. The (3-9)heptapeptide fragment of [D-Ser(Bu^t)^6] LH-RH(1-9)EA did not show pituitary accumulation, even though it had some residual LH releasing activity.
It is concluded, that pituitary accumulation of labelled LH-RH analogues and biological activity are well correlated, highly active analogues being bound to the pituitary for considerably longer periods than LH-RH.

Hoechst AG., 623 Frankfurt 80, Pharmacology H 821

174

STUDIES ON THE MECHANISM OF ACTION OF THE ISOPRENALINE-INDUCED INCREASE IN PLASMA CONCENTRATIONS OF VASOPRESSIN IN THE RAT.   W. Knepel and D.K. Meyer

The ß-sympathomimetic amine isoprenaline (given i.m. or s.c.) causes antidiuresis. This renal effect of the amine has been shown to depend on an intact neurohypophysis, i.e. on the release and action of antidiuretic hormone (ADH) (Schrier et al., J.Clin.Invest. 51,97,1972). Using a sensitive and specific radioimmunoassay for the determination of ADH the effect of i.m. injections of isoprenaline on the plasma levels of the peptide was investigated in rats.

Isoprenaline caused a dose- and time-dependent increase in plasma concentrations of ADH. The role in the isoprenaline-induced secretion of ADH of some parameters, which are known to regulate ADH-release was investigated. Plasma osmolality and blood volume were not changed after administration of isoprenaline. However, dehydration potentiated the effect of isoprenaline on ADH-release, while previous hydration of the rats abolished it. There was a correlation of the blood pressure lowering effect of the amine with its action ADH-release. The involvement of the renin angiotensin system was also tested. Saralasin, a competitive antagonist of angiotensin II, had no clear-cut effect on the isoprenaline-induced ADH-release, when it was infused intravenously.

It is concluded that the ß-sympathomimetic amine causes the release of ADH mainly by its blood pressure lowering effect. Other parameters which are known to be in control of ADH-release seem to be of minor or no importance.

Department of Pharmacology, University of Freiburg, Hermann-Herder-Strasse 5, D-7800 Freiburg i.Br.

175

Specific Binding of [^{125}J]insulin to Isolated Pancreatic Islets of Rats and Its Relationship to Glucose Metabolism   E.J. Verspohl, and H.P.T.Ammon

Exogenous insulin has been shown to decrease islet pentosephosphate shunt (PPS) activity, NADPH/NADP ratio and glucose induced insulin release. It was now studied whether insulin specifically binds to pancreatic islets and whether or not such a binding correlates with insulin induced changes of islet metabolism.
Collagenase isolated islets were incubated with [^{125}J]insulin in KRB-albumin buffer. After filtering the radioactivity of islets was counted. Binding of [^{125}J]insulin was total binding corrected for unspecific binding (adding 1 U/ml of unlabelled insulin).
Binding linearly depends on the number of islets. Binding is a saturable process with respect to time (maximum after 20 min) as well as with respect to insulin (4.5 µU/250 islets at a concentration of 800 uU/ml). Plotting the results in a Scatchard plot, the number of binding sites is about 1.1x10^8/1 islet. Native insulin competes with [^{125}J]insulin for binding in a dose-dependent manner (K_d = 160 µU/ml). A similar K_d (150 µU/ml) was found incubating islets with [^{125}J]insulin. When the insulin (0, 200, 400, 800 µU/ml) induced decrease of islet PPS activity, 6PG/G6P ratio, NADPH/NADP ratio and glucose stimulated insulin release as observed in earlier studies (Endocrinology 99, 1469 (1976); Diabetes 26, 857 (1977)) is plotted against the binding of [^{125}J]insulin to pancreatic islets a close relationship was obvious.
Conclusion. 1.Our data strongly suggest a specific binding of insulin to pancreatic rat islets. 2. Specific binding correlates with insulin induced changes of islet metabolism.

Department of Pharmacology, Institute of Pharmaceutical Sciences, University D-74 Tuebingen, Auf der Morgenstelle

176

IS STIMULATION OF GLUCOSE METABOLISM NECESSARY FOR INITIATION OF INSULIN RELEASE?   S. Holze, U. Panten

Glucose is the major physiological stimulus for insulin secretion but there are some other substances which can initiate insulin release as well. ∝-ketoisocaproic acid (∝-KIC) has turned out to be the most potent of them. It was shown that glucose induced insulin release is always accompanied by an enhancement of glucose metabolism by the ß-cells but it has remained unsettled whether the stimulation of glucose metabolism is indispensable to initiate insulin secretion. To get more information on this point we investigated whether or not glucose metabolism is stimulated when insulin release is induced by an initiator other than glucose.
Isolated islets of obese hyperglycemic mice were incubated in a small volume of medium supplemented with low and high concentrations of 5-^{3}H-glucose in the absence and presence of ∝-KIC which was shown to induce a marked increase in insulin release in our incubation system. Glucose metabolism was calculated from T$_2$O formation from 5-^{3}H-glucose.
In the presence of ∝-KIC glucose metabolic rates were never found to be enhanced.
Our results showing that induction of insulin release by ∝-KIC is not accompanied by an increase in glucose metabolism indicate that initiation of insulin release must not necessarily be mediated by stimulation of glucose metabolism.

Institute of Pharmacology and Toxicology, University of Göttingen, Robert-Koch-Str. 40, D-3400 Göttingen

177

INFLUENCE OF SORBITOL AND MANNITOL ON THE INHI-
BITORY EFFECT OF ALLOXAN ON INSULIN RELEASE BY
PANCREATIC ISLETS   J. Beckmann, H.-J. Goldberg

The mechanism by which glucose (G) prevents ß-
cell-destruction by alloxan (A) is not settled.
Since it had been shown that the sugar alcohols
sorbitol (S) and mannitol (M) though not stimulating the ß-cells by themselves enhance the G-
induced insulin release (IR), the question arose
whether these polyols, which also had been shown
not to diminish A-toxicity in the absence of G,
might increase ß-cell-protection by G as well.
Isolated mouse islets were preincubated for 20
min with 17mM S, 8.8mM G, 8.8mM G + 17mM S, or
8.8mM G + 17mM M. A (1mM final conc.) was then
added and after 20 min. the medium was changed
and the islets incubated for 60 min. in the presence of 16.7mM G. IR during this period was the
parameter of residual ß-cell-activity.
Preincubation with S alone had no, 8.8mM G alone
only a small protective effect. Relative rates
of IR after preincubation with G, G + S, and G
+ M resp. were 1 : 2.33 : 1.40. It is thus shown
that S and M, though not lowering A-toxicity by
themselves, analogue to their action on IR can
nevertheless enhance ß-cell-protection by G.
Since M cannot be transported and metabolized by
the ß-cell the process of protection seems to be
independent of transport- and metabolic events
and to take place at the plasma membrane.

Institute of Pharmacology and Toxicology,
University of Göttingen, Robert-Koch-Str. 40
D 3400 Göttingen

178

THE INSULIN RELEASING POTENCY OF TOLBUTAMIDE AND
GLIBENCLAMIDE: A COMPARATIVE STUDY ON THE PER-
FUSED RAT PANCREAS.
H.G. Joost

Glibenclamide, the "second generation" sulfonylurea, stimulates insulin release at much smaller
concentrations than tolbutamide. Moreover, differences of the kinetic pattern and the dynamics of
insulin release have been assumed. The experimental observations that suggested qualitative differences, however, seemed not completely convin-
cing. Thus the effects of the sulfonylurea derivatives on the isolated perfused rat pancreas
were compared, an in vitro system well suited to
study both kinetics and dynamics of insulin release.
In the presence of 7.5 mM glucose both sulfonylurea derivatives produced the same secretion
pattern: An overshooting peak was followed by an
elevated stable plateau of insulin release. Further, the quantity of the effect closely depended
on the glucose concentration: The compounds stimulated maximally at 7.5 and 10 mM glucose. No
additional insulin release by sulfonylurea could
be observed at 20 and 30 mM glucose indicating
that the dose response curve had been shifted to
lower glucose concentrations. There was no difference between tolbutamide and glibenclamide except for the concentration of sulfonylurea needed. In conclusion: Tolbutamide and glibenclamide enhance the responsiveness of the ß-cell
to glucose but do not alter the maximal secretion. No evidence for qualitative differences
between the two "generations" of sulfonylurea
derivatives could be provided by our in vitro
model.
Institute of Pharmacology and Toxicology,
University of Göttingen, Robert-Koch-Straße 40,
D 3400 Göttingen

179

Insulin Secretion and Metabolism of Pancreatic
Islets from ob/ob Mice after Thyroxine Treatment
S. Lenzen

Thyroxine treatment (2000 ug/kg b.wt., for 5
days) induced experimental hyperthyroidism in
ob/ob mice. The relation between insulin secretion and metabolism of pancreatic islets was investigated. Thyroxine treatment inhibited glucose-
induced insulin secretion from the isolated perfused ob/ob mouse pancreas and reduced total pancreas insulin content. Histological examination
of the pancreas revealed islets with well preserved beta cells which appeared to be reduced in
size but not in number. Quantitative evaluation
showed a decrease of the beta cell area in relation to the total pancreatic parenchyma probably
due to reduced islet cell volume. Glucose-induced
insulin release from incubated pancreatic islets
and insulin content of pancreatic islets were not
reduced after thyroxine treatment. ATP content of
islets was normal. Glucose oxidation and glucose
utilization by islets were increased. Thyroxine
treatment suppressed potentiation of glucose-induced $^{45}Ca^{2+}$ uptake into the lantanum-nondis-
placeable pool of islets induced by fasting in
control mice.
The metabolic characteristics of pancreatic islets from ob/ob mice after thyroxine treatment
are those of all hyperthyroid tissues, representing an increased rather than a decreased metabolic activity. The results provide no evidence
for a disturbed metabolic function or energy de-
priviation of pancreatic islets. Inhibition of insulin secretion from the pancreas seems to be due
to a reduction in total pancreas insulin content
and a reduced pancreatic islet volume.

Institute of Pharmacology and Toxicology,
University of Göttingen, Robert-Koch-Str. 40,
D-3400 Göttingen

180

PHARMACODYNAMIC EFFECTS OF LITHOSPERMUM OFFICINALE ON THE
METABOLISM OF THYROID HORMONES IN THE RAT
H. Winterhoff, H. Sourgens, F. H. Kemper, F. Aenstoots

The antithyroid properties of Lithospermum officinale
which had been investigated in the guinea pig, were confirmed in the rat. Serum hormone levels of thyroxine and
triiodothyronine and the secretion rate (endocytosis)
were examined. Several sites of action are discussed.

The single intravenous injection of Lithospermum officinale freeze dried extract (FDE) incubated with 1 IU TSH
resulted in a fall of the thyroid hormones concentration
under control levels, the decline is even more pronounced
when Lithospermum FDE is injected alone. The duration and
degree of secretion is clearly reduced in the TSH and
Lithospermum FDE-treated animals as compared to the
hormone treated control rats, whereas Lithospermum alone
suppressed even the basal secretion, which can be monitored in saline injected control rats.

These results were compared as well with the effects of
KI, a known inhibitor of thyroidal secretion, as KI + TSH.
Thyroid hormone levels declined more rapidly and several
hours earlier in the TSH and Lithospermum FDE-treated
rats than in TSH and KI-treated animals, despite of
maximal KI-dosage.

The decline of triiodothyronine concentrations to un-
measurable levels in Lithospermum FDE-injected animals
may be partly due to a peripheral site of action. In
thyroidectomized thyroxine substituted rats T_3-levels
were reduced significantly by intravenous injection of
Lithospermum FDE.

Institute of Pharmacology and Toxicology, University of
Münster, Westring 12, D-44oo Münster

181

NUTRITIONAL FACTORS STIMULATING GASTRIC MUCOSAL DNA AND RNA SYNTHESIS. D. Müller and K.-Fr. Sewing

In starved animals gastric mucosal DNA and RNA synthesis can be stimulated by gastrin and pentagastrin (L.R.Johnson, Gastroenterology $\underline{70}$, 278, 1976). Gastrin is much less active than refeeding in restoring DNA and RNA synthesis. It was the purpose of the present study to search for nutritional factors stimulating gastric mucosal DNA and RNA synthesis. The experiments were carried out in female rats which were killed 16 hrs after the normal pellet food was withdrawn and replaced by food mixtures. DNA synthesis was measured by incorporation of ^{3}H-thymidine, and RNA synthesis by incorporation of ^{3}H-uridine. Data were normalized as percent of control (normal food). 16 hrs starvation reduced DNA synthesis by 77.5+5% and RNA synthesis by 95.5+1%. The effect of various compositions (Food mixture in % (w/w): peptone 28.6, carbohydrates 28.6, Psyllium 28.6, olive oil 14.2, C-food mixture:peptone 14.3, carbohydrates 14.3, olive oil 14.2, cellulose 57.2) are summarized in the table.

	DNA	RNA
		synthesis (in %)
Normally fed	100	100
Starved for 16 hrs	22.5+ 5.0	4.5+ 1
Food mixture	54.6+19.8	24.0+11.6$^+$
Food mixture+3 % Na$_2$HPO$_4$	91.6+10.6$^+$	44.6+ 5.9$^+$
Food mixture+3 % NaCl	67.0+22.2$^+$	38.7+14.6$^+$
Food mixture+3 % KCl	81.3+26.1$^+$	26.2+ 9.6$^+$
C-food mixture	73.3+14.2$^+$	20.8+ 4.6$^+$

$^+$significantly different from starved animals (p at least <0.05).
DNA synthesis is less susceptible than RNA synthesis to starvation but more susceptible to feeding. Additional Na$_2$HPO$_4$ or KCl almost completely prevents the drop in DNA synthesis. Obviously none of the mixtures counteracted the effect of starvation on RNA synthesis completely. Further research for specific nutritional stimulatory factors is necessary.

Department of Pharmacology, University of Tübingen, D 7400 Tübingen, Wilhelmstr. 56

182

H-SECRETION - A DRIVING FORCE IN NACL ABSORPTION OF THE GUINEA PIG GALLBLADDER K.-U. Petersen and K. Heintze

The absorption of Na and Cl in the gallbladder of the guinea pig is partly dependent on the HCO$_3$ in the bathing medium (D.W.Martin, J.Membrane Biol., 18, 219, 1974; J. Wood et al.,Pflügers Arch., $\underline{365}$, R15, 1976). To elucidate the nature of this HCO$_3$-effect we measured net volume fluxes and the net fluxes of Na, Cl and H. The alkalination of the mucosal side in HCO$_3$-buffered solutions, due to a Cl-HCO$_3$ exchange (K. Heintze et al., Naunyn Schmiedebergs Arch. Pharm., $\underline{297}$, R38, 1977), was reversed into an acidification, if HCO$_3$ was omitted. In this HCO$_3$-free solution luminal pH and the fluid absorption decreased within 40 min exponentially to a final pH of 6.5$\pm$0.05 and an absorption rate of 6.7$\pm$1.6 μl·cm^{-2}·hr^{-1} respectively. The time courses of luminal acidification and of fluid absorption in PO$_4$-buffered and in HCO$_3$-free salines were identical whereas the luminal pH after 40 min was 7.2$\pm$0.01 in the PO$_4$-buffered group. Hence the decline of fluid absorption was probably not due to a limiting H-gradient. Neither Tris nor pyruvate nor glycodiazine could mimic the absorption stimulating effect of HCO$_3$ but butyrate concentration dependently restored net fluid and Na absorption. 25 mM butyrate were equieffective to 25 mM HCO$_3$. Formiate (no effect), acetate, propionate and butyrate were increasingly effective in stimulating fluid absorption. Both butyrate and HCO$_3$ are likely to combine with a secreted H to form lipid soluble molecule in the lumen of the gallbladder.

Department of Pharmacology, RWTH Aachen, Melatenerstr. 213, D-5100 Aachen.

183

COMPOSITION AND LITHOGENITY OF BILE IN RATS AND DOGS AFTER LONG TERM APPLICATION OF CLANOBUTIN J. Schlepper, E. Kraas, and R. Gastauer

The effect of clanobutin (4[p-chloro-N-(p-methoxyphenyl-) benzamido]butyric acid), on secretion and lithogenity of bile under long term application was studied in conscious rats and dogs. Although bile composition in rats and dogs are not identical with that in man at least predictions are allowed about the effect on human bile.
Bile was collected by implanted tubes in a system allowing a continuous flow to the duodenum. Samples were taken from fed rats (16 hours after clanobutin) and from fed dogs (90 min after clanobutin, 30 min after nutritive stimulation) and from the same dogs after 22.5 hours fasting (16 hours after clanobutin, pancreozymin stimulated). Rats were given 200 mg/kg clanobutin p.o. daily for 10 days. Dogs were treated over a fortnight with 50 mg/kg p.o. twice a day. Data were compared intraindividually in dogs and interindividually in rats.
In both species clanobutin caused a bile salt independent choleretic effect. It is mainly eliminated biliary as an organic anion in both species. In rats the volume of bile secretion was significantly increased while the output of bile acids, cholesterol and phospholipids remained unaltered. In the same rats the pancreatic secretion of protein was stimulated up to 190 % without any change in pancreatic flow. In dogs bile flow and output of Na$^+$ and K$^+$ were significantly increased. Concentrations of phospholipids and cholesterol were significantly reduced in fed and fasted dogs. Bile acids were reduced also but to a less extend. Therefore the lithogenic index was diminished significantly.

Byk Gulden Lomberg Chemische Fabrik GmbH, Forschungslaboratorien, Byk-Gulden-Str. 2, D 7750 Konstanz

184

EFFECTS OF POLYUNSATURATED FATTY ACIDS ON GASTRIC SECRETION IN RATS H. Vapaatalo, J. Parantainen, T. Metsä-Ketelä, and K. Keyriläinen

Prostaglandins (PGs) regulate many functions of the gastro-intestinal tract. PGE and PGA inhibit gastric secretion stimulated by various agents in different animal species (cf. A. Robert, Proc. Sixth Int. Congr. Pharmacol. $\underline{5}$, 161, 1975). Less is known about the actions of PG-precursors on gastric secretion. In the present study the effects of arachidonic acid (AA) and linolic acid (LA) were studied on pentagastrin-stimulated gastric secretion in the rat. Fasted male rats were urethane-anaesthetized and their stomachs perfused continuously with saline (0.8 ml/min). Samples were collected for 5 min, and H$^+$ was titrated. Pentagastrin-infusion (1.2 µg/kg/min) increased the acid secretion 6- to 10-fold. The steady state was reached in about 30 min. Thereafter AA- (100 µg/kg/min) or LA- (400 µg/kg/min) infusion was started with continued pentagastrin-administration. In about 30 min the acid secretion was reduced near to the basal level by AA. LA strongly potentiated the pentagastrin-stimulated acid output.
It can be suggested that AA inhibits the acid secretion by acting as a PG-precursor. The increase in the acid secretion by LA might be due to the competitive inhibition of prostaglandin cyclo-oxygenase.

Grant: Orion and Medica Scientific Foundation, Finland

Department of Biomedical Sciences, University of Tampere, Box 607, SF-33101 Tampere 10, Finland

185

PGE-MEDIATED EFFECT OF DIPHENOLIC LAXATIVES
E. Beubler and H. Juan

Diphenolic laxatives such as phenolphthalein (P) and bisacodyl (B) and PGE inhibit absorption and increase secretion of water and electrolytes in the gut. We investigated whether B and P exert their action via stimulation of PGE biosynthesis in the gut. B and P were compared with the osmotic laxatives mannitol, 4 % (M) and Na_2SO_4, 3. 85 % (N).

The influence of the laxatives was tested: (1) on water net flux in the tied off colon of the rat in situ in controls and after inhibition of PG release by pretreatment with indomethacin, (2) on water net flux and on PGE release in the perfused colon (3) on intestinal blood flow in jejunal loops in situ.

In the tied off colon, B (1 and 10 µg/ml) and P (10 and 100 µg/ml) dose dependently increased water net flux toward the lumen (p < 0.01). Indomethacin reduced the effect of B and P (p < 0.05). The osmotic laxatives M and N also increased water net flux towards the lumen (p < 0.01). However, this effect was not reduced by indomethacin.

In the perfused colon all the laxatives tested also increased water net flux towards the lumen. B (10 and 50 µg/ml) and P (100 and 500 µg/ml) dose dependently (p < 0.02) stimulated the release of PGE into the gut lumen. M and N did not stimulate PGE release.

In jejunal loops of the rat in situ B (100 µg/ml) increased intestinal blood flow by 50 % (p < 0.01). This effect was inhibited by indomethacin (p < 0.01).

It is concluded that diphenolic laxatives exert their effect via stimulation of biosynthesis of PGE in the gut.

Institut für Experimentelle und Klinische Pharmakologie
Universitätsplatz 4, A-8010 G r a z

186

EFFECTS OF CHOLINERGIC STIMULATION ON ISOLATED MAST CELLS FROM RAT, GUINEA PIG AND MAN
G. Poblete-Freundt, C. Rauch, W. Schönfeld, and W. Schmutzler

Acetylcholine (Ach) in a certain concentration range has been reported to augment the allergic release of mediator substances from human lung (Kaliner et al., J.exp.Med.,136,556,1972). In the perfused guinea pig lung Ach (10^{-8} M) exerted a rather inhibitory effect on the allergic histamine release (Gesener et al., Atemw.Lung.Kr.,3, 13,1977). However, in nonsensitized rat mast cells Ach itself ($>10^{-11}$ M) caused a strong histamine release (Fantozzi et al., Agents Actions, in press).
In our present experiments occurred a striking difference in the behaviour of isolated mast cells from sensitized or nonsensitized individuals. Ach (10^{-10}-10^{-6} M) caused in human mast cells a dosage dependent histamine release if the cells were capable to react to anti-human-IgE. However, Ach had dual, enhancing and inhibiting effects on the anti-human-IgE induced histamine release itself.
In nonsensitized guinea pig mast cells Ach or carbachol were ineffective. However, Ach (10^{-8} - 10^{-6} M) caused a strong histamine release if the cells were isolated from actively sensitized tissues. If these cells were challenged with Ach and antigen simultaneously the allergic histamine release was inhibited at Ach 10^{-12}, 10^{-10} or 10^{-6} M but increased at Ach 10^{-8} M.
The results support the hypothesis (Behrendt, in press) based on ultrastructural evidence that sensitization increases the susceptibility of mast cells for cell function modulating influences.

Department of Pharmacology, Medical Faculty, RWTH Aachen, Melatenerstr. 213, D-5100 Aachen.

187

INHIBITION OF COMPLEMENT ACTIVATION BY THE CHEMO-TACTIC DRUG, PROPAMIDINE   W. Vogt

Propamidine is one out of several diamidines used as chemotherapeutic drugs against infections with Babesiae and Leishmaniae. It binds to the third component of complement (C3) and inhibits complement-dependent immune haemolysis (Ashgar and Cormane, Immunochemistry 13, 975, 1976). A detailed analysis shows that mainly two steps of the complement reaction are inhibited: activation of the fourth (C4) and fifth (C5) components. An inhibition of C5 activation was anticipated since surface-fixed C3b (the fragment representing the activated form of C3) is essential for C5 activation and fulfils its function only when free of other potential ligands (Vogt et al., Immunology 34, 1978). Interference with C4 and C5 activation means an inhibition of cytotoxic effects of complement, while activation by the alternative pathway up to the step of C3 utilization is still possible. Hence, some complement effects - opsonization, phagocytosis, release of the biologically active peptide C3a - should be able to proceed in the presence of propamidine. Possibly the anticomplementary effects of propamidine are related to its chemotherapeutic action since Babesiae enter red cells only when an intact complement system is present (Chapman and Ward, Science 196, 67 (1977).

Max-Planck-Institut für experimentelle Medizin, Department of Biochemical Pharmacology, Hermann-Rein-Str. 3, 3400 Göttingen, Germany.

188

AGGREGATION OF LEUKOCYTES BY NATURAL AND SYNTHETIC CHEMOTACTIC PEPTIDES   B. Damerau

Several chemotactic factors which induce directed migration of leukocytes in vitro (Boyden chamber) also caused aggregation of human blood leukocytes. The cells were separated by sedimentation of blood in a dextran-containing medium, suspended in Gey's solution with 0.5 % human serum albumin to a final concentration of 10^7 cells/ml and incubated with continuous stirring at 37^0 C in an aggregometer. All chemotactic factors investigated showed this effect: The cleavage peptides from the third and fifth component of hog complement, C3a and C5a, and the synthetic formyl-peptides f-met-leu-OH, f-met-leu-leu-OH and f-met-leu-phe-OH. The aggregation was dose-dependent and occurred only in the presence of both Mg^{++} and Ca^{++}. Further details were studied with C5a and f-met-leu-phe-OH. Leukocytes incubated in Ca^{++}- and Mg^{++}-free medium with these peptides were specifically desensitized. Aggregation was totally inhibited by the SH-reagent N-ethylmaleimide (0.1 mM), but only partly by p-chloromercuribenzoate (0.1 mM). Inhibition was also caused by the chymotrypsin inhibitor tosyl-lysyl-chloromethyl-ketone (but not by the esterase substrates BAEE and TAME) and by colchicine (3 and 10 µg/ml). In contrast the microfilament desintegrating agent cytochalasin B (0.4 and 2.0 µg/ml) greatly enhanced aggregation by the peptides.

Max-Planck-Institut für experimentelle Medizin, Department of Biochemical Pharmacology, Hermann-Rein-Str. 3, D-3400 Göttingen, Germany.

189

INITIATION AND MODULATION OF ECF GENERATION AND SECRETION FROM HUMAN POLYMORPHONUCLEAR NEUTRO-PHILS[x]. W. König, H. Tesch and N. Frickhofen

The primary mediators which are involved in inflammatory processes are histamine, the slow reacting substance of anaphylaxis (SRS-A), the platelet aggregating factor (PAF) and the eosinophil chemotactic factor (ECF). These mediators are primarily localized within mast cells and basophil leucocytes, which represent the target cells of allergic reaction. Binding of IgE to mast cells and basophil leucocytes and addition of the appropriate antigen then leads to the activation of the target cells with a subsequent release of their mediators. SRS and ECF have also been found in a non mast cell source, e.g. in human PMNs. ECF can be generated and released from human PMNs by different stimuli, such as the Ca ionophore, antigen antibody complexes and arachidonic acid. The generation of ECF is dose-, time- and temperature-dependent. In each case a low molecular weight mediator (500 daltons) is released which specifically attracts guinea pig or human eosinophils in a modified Boyden chamber. The secretion of ECF is modulated by agents affecting the cyclic nucleotide level within PMNs or by antiphlogistic substances, while ECF itself is inactivated by serum and cell derived factors. The latter inactivator is present within the granules of PMNs. We conclude that various stimuli attract eosinophils to sites of inflammation where they counteract inflammatory reactions.

x Supported by DFG, SFB 107, A6

Department of Medical Microbiology, Johannes Gutenberg-University, 6500 Mainz, Germany

190

INHIBITION OF THE ANTIAGGREGATORY ACTIVITY OF THE VESSEL WALL (RAT) BY ACETYLSALICYLIC ACID
F. Seuter, W.D. Busse, and W. Gau

The antiaggregatory activity of the vessel wall (rat) and its inhibition by acetylsalicylic acid(ASA) was tested under different experimental conditions (dose- and time related effects) in human platelet rich plasma (BORN-techn.):

Time interval after oral administration	Tris-buffer	Tragac.-Control	mg/kg orally ASA		
			3	1o	3o
9o min					
Sham operation	1oo+2	12 + 4	23+8	63+ 5*	97+4*
Chilling of the vessel **	1oo+2	1o + 3	34+9*	62+12*	95+5*
24 h					
Sham operation	1oo+2	8 + 2	25+6*	51+11*	83+4*
Chilling of the vessel **	1oo+2	7 + 1	32+8*	35+1o*	73+9*

*= significant with p < o.o5 (control vs. ASA)
**= under the conditions of exper.induced thrombosis (1)

As indicated in the table the antiaggregatory activity of the vessel wall is inhibited by ASA in a dose-dependent manner. In order to examine, whether these effects are due to prostacyclin (PGI 2)-generation or ADP'ase activity the latter was determined in preparations of the carotid artery by a new procedure for analysis of ADP degradation products (adenine nucleotides) utilizing high pressure liquid chromatography. Its activity was not influenced by ASA (1oo mg/kg orally). It is postulated that PGI 2 synthesis of the vessel wall is mediated by a specific cyclooxygenase similar to that of the platelet membranes which is blocked by ASA in vivo. The relevance of these data regarding the formation of thrombi is difficult to judge, because ASA has already been shown to be an effective antithrombotic drug (1) in the same dose range as mentioned above.

(1) = Meng/Seuter: Naun.Schmied.Arch.Pharmacol.(in press).
Institute of Pharmacology, BAYER AG, D-56oo Wuppertal 1, Postfach 1o17o9

191

EXPERIMENTAL OSTEOARTHROSIS FOR PHARMACOLOGICAL ANTI-ARTHROTIC COMPOUNDS

by D.A. Kalbhen

Using adult hens as laboratory animals we found that 2 intraarticular injections of 0,25 mg or 0,5 mg iodo-acetate into the knee joint can induce experimental osteoarthrosis within a period of 2-3 months. By macroscopical, histological and biochemical criteria the slowly progressing degenerations in the joint are in good correlation with human osteoarthrosis. In pharmacological experiments we tried to inhibit the degenerative processes in our model of osteoarthrosis by treatment with natural and semisynthetic acidic polysaccharides: pentosan polysulfate (SP-54), DAK-16 (from Rumalon[R]) and a mucopolysaccharide polysulfate (Arteparon[R]). After weekly intraarticular applications of these compounds in a dose range of 0,001 mg - 0,1 mg per injection a significant anti-arthrotic potency could be demonstrated, while higher doses had no or an adverse effect.

As seen in the living animal by special X-ray technique and by measurements of joint space, the tested drugs are able to slow down and to inhibit the progressing osteoarthrosis. After autopsy and preparation of the knee joints our results from X-ray investigations were confirmed by macroscopic evaluation of the articular cartilage. Since degenerative processes in articular connective tissue involve the participation of catabolic (lysosomal) enzymes, the anti-arthrotic effect of the tested drugs: pentosane polysulfate, DAK-16, and Arteparon[R] can be explained by their potency to inhibit proteases and mucopolysaccharidases (glycosaminoglycan hydrolases).

Pharmakologisches Institut der Universität Bonn, Reuterstrasse 2 b, 53 Bonn, West-Germany

192

ION-DEPENDENCE OF ATP-STIMULATED LYSIS OF CHROMAFFIN GRANULES   A. Burger and M. Castritius

ATP-Mg^{++} stimulates osmotic lysis of chromaffin granules, which are suspended in an isotonic medium containing NaCl or KCl. Attempting to elucidate this process we examined some anions and cations for ATP-stimulated swelling of chromaffin granules from bovine adrenals by measuring the optical density at 430nm during 40min at 20°C. The cuvettes contained granules (appr. 90µg protein) suspended in 2ml 30mM Tris-Hepes (pH 7.4), 3mM ATP-Mg^{++} (controls: only Mg^{++}), solutes and sucrose to achieve 300mOsm. In the following sequence of potency 40mM K$^+$-salts caused swelling: Br$^-$ ≃ Cl$^-$ < SCN$^-$ ≃ NO$_3^-$ ≃ ClO$_3^-$ ≃ I$^-$ < ClO$_4^-$, which was stimulated by ATP. Acetate, citrate, phosphate and sulfate (up to 100mM Na$^+$- or K$^+$-salts) showed no effects. In samples with 100mM K$^+$-salts valinomycin (1µg/ml) caused faster swelling than ATP, the sequence of potency being the same except SCN$^-$, which was the most potent anion with valinomycin. The stimulating effects of ATP were inhibited by DCCD, NEM, DNP, antimycin A, rotenone or by an hypertonic medium. ATP stimulated the swelling more with 136mM K$^+$-salts of Cl$^-$, Br$^-$, NO$_3^-$ and ClO$_3^-$ than with Na$^+$-salts. From different chlorides (40-136mM) the following cations showed ATP-effects: Choline < Tris ≃ Na$^+$ < Li$^+$ ≃ K$^+$. Mg^{++}-salts (35mM) induced shrinkage of granules, which was enhanced in the absence of ATP: Cl$^-$ > NO$_3^-$ > ClO$_4$. NH$_4^+$-salts and urea evoked a rapid ATP-independent lysis of granules. Concluding hypothesis: At the granular membrane ATP-hydrolysis supports an inward-directed translocation of protons, which allow the exchange against some monovalent cations like K$^+$. As a result of the electrochemical gradient anions which can penetrate the membrane in the non-protonated form follow the entry of cations. Water follows the solutes and induces swelling and finally disruption of the granules.

Dept. of Pharmacology, University of Würzburg

193

ROLE OF NERVE GROWTH FACTOR IN THE FUNCTION OF SYMPATHETIC NEURONS AND ADRENAL MEDULLARY CELLS. Otten,U., Goedert,M. and Thoenen,H.

Administration of nerve growth factor (NGF) to newborn and adult rats leads to a selective induction of tyrosine hydroxylase (TH) and dopamine ß-hydroxylase (DBH) in sympathetic ganglia and adrenal medullae.
Neutralization of endogenous NGF or cross reacting NGF-like molecules by antibodies leads to a distinct impairment of the synthesis of the adrenergic transmitter, norepinephrine. Administration of monospecific anti NGF-antibodies results in an irreversible, drastic reduction in TH, DBH and dopa decarboxylase in sympathetic ganglia of newborn rats. In contrast, the enzyme reduction in adult animals is smaller and reversible. The shift from the irreversible to the reversible effect is a gradual one. Administration of anti NGF-antibodies on day 2 and 6 after birth leads to an irreversible effect. At day 12 the effect is partially and at day 16 fully reversible.
The fact that immunization of adult rats against NGF also reduced all catecholamine-synthesizing enzymes indicates that NGF is not only essential for the development of the peripheral sympathetic nervous system but also for the maintenance of its function after differentiation.

Dept. of Pharmacology, Biocenter of the University, Basel, Switzerland

This work was supported by the Swiss National Foundation for Scientific Research (Grant Nr. 3.432.74).

194

CHANGES OF DOPAMINE-ß-HYDROXYLASE ACTIVITY IN HUMAN PLASMA DURING PROLONGED OVERACTIVITY OF THE SYMPATHETIC NERVOUS SYSTEM IN VARIOUS DISEASES. A.F.Hammerle, H.Hörtnagl, R.Stadler-Wolffersgrün, Th.Brücke, and J.M.Hackl

For the evaluation of dopamine-ß-hydroxylase (DBH) activity in plasma as an index of the sympathetic nervous system mainly experiments with acute stimulation of the sympathetic nervous system have been performed. However little is known about the changes of DBH activity in plasma at occasions of prolonged overactivity of the sympathetic nervous system. We have therefore estimated adrenaline, noradrenaline and DBH activity in plasma of 10 patients (with head injury, tetanus and fat embolism syndrome) with clinical symptoms indicative of sympathetic overactivity which lasted for several days or even weeks. It could be demonstrated that long-lasting increases of catecholamine levels in plasma were accompanied by a gradual decline of DBH activity. The decrease of DBH activity in plasma was more pronounced in those patients with especially high plasma catecholamine levels. In 3 patients only 13 % to 16 % of the initial DBH activity remained after an increase in the activity of the sympathetic nervous system lasting 3 to 4 weeks.
Four patients suffering from head injury without signs of an overactivity of the sympathetic nervous system did not show a decrease of DBH activity in plasma. From these and previous data reported in the literature it is suggested that plasma DBH activity is not an useful index of the sympatho-adrenal activity in a situation of longlasting overactivity.

Department of Pharmacology, University of Innsbruck, A-6020 Innsbruck, Peter Mayr Straße 1

195

EXERCISE INDUCED CHANGES OF CATECHOLAMINES AND POTASSIUM IN PLASMA AFTER TREATMENT WITH PROPRANOLOL IN DOGS
E. Appel, F. Starey[*], H. Grobecker, E. Lindner[*], A.H. Staib, H. Grötsch[*]

Previous studies in man have shown that during ß-adrenoceptor blockade physical exercise caused a significantly greater elevation of plasma catecholamines than without blockade. After blockade of ß-adrenoceptors, increased levels of circulating catecholamines should have an unopposed effect on adrenergic α-receptors. In order to elucidate such an effect, experiments were performed on 7 trained dogs before and after ß-adrenoceptor blockade (0.1 mg/kg (-)-propranolol i.v.). Exercise was performed on a conveyor (10 min, 10 km/h, slope 10%). Besides catecholamine concentrations in plasma as an index of α-receptor agonism plasma K^+ was determined (Castro-Tavares, Arzneim.Forsch. 26, 238, 1976). Directly after exercise, plasma noradrenaline was increased from 310 to 461 ng/l, plasma adrenaline from 172 to 222 ng/l and plasma potassium from 4.23 to 4.6 mmol/l. After ß-adrenoceptor blockade exercise caused a significantly higher increase in plasma noradrenaline (569 ng/l) and plasma adrenaline (260 ng/l). Also plasma potassium concentrations were significantly elevated (5.05 mmol/l). - The results indicate a reflex activation of sympatho-neuronal and sympatho-adrenal mechanisms during exercise after ß-adrenoceptor blockade, leading to a reduced ß-receptor blockade and a pronounced stimulation of α-adrenoceptors.

Departments of Pharmacology, University of Frankfurt/Main and Farbwerke Hoechst AG[*]

196

THE INFLUENCE OF THE RATE OF PERFUSION ON THE KINETICS OF NEURONAL UPTAKE IN THE RABBIT ISOLATED HEART
K.-H. Graefe and B. Keller

Reserpine-pretreated rabbit hearts (the MAO and COMT of which were inhibited) were perfused at rates ranging from 1.3 to 11.3 ml·g^{-1}·min^{-1} with ^{14}C-sorbitol and various concentrations (0.4 - 20 /uM) of ^{3}H-(-)noradrenaline (NA). From measurements of the arterio-venous concentration difference of ^{3}H and ^{14}C activity the removal of NA and sorbitol from the perfusion fluid was followed for 2-3 min at intervals of 5 s. The uptake of NA into intracellular spaces of the heart (proved to be overwhelmingly into sympathetic nerve terminals) was obtained by subtraction of the removal of sorbitol from that of NA; it was cumulated and plotted against time. In this way progress curves of NA uptake were constructed in each experiment. Following a brief lag period, these curves exhibited a linear phase of uptake. From the slope of the linear phase initial rates of NA uptake were obtained.
At any given rate of perfusion, the initial rates of NA uptake obeyed Michaelis-Menten kinetics. While changes of the perfusion rate did not alter the apparent K_m (range: 2.2 - 2.4 /uM), a rectangular hyperbolic relationship was found between V_{max} and the rate of perfusion. The V_{max} was half-maximal at a flow rate of 2.7 ml·g^{-1}·min^{-1} and approached a maximum value of 9.0 nmoles·g^{-1}·min^{-1}. The lack of change of the K_m indicates that the uptake sites of the heart are functionally arranged in parallel, whereas the change in V_{max} implies that their accessibility is dependent on the flow rate. (Supported by the DFG)

Department of Pharmacology, University of Würzburg, Versbacher Landstrasse 9, D-8700 Würzburg

197

CONTRIBUTION BY NEURONAL AND EXTRANEURONAL MECHANISMS TO
THE ELIMINATION OF NORADRENALINE FROM THE EXTRACELLULAR
SPACE (RABBIT AORTA)   M. Henseling

For the inactivation of exogenous noradrenaline (NA)
neuronal uptake and extraneuronal O-methylation represent
the two functionally important mechanisms.

To determine K_m and V_{max} for the neuronal uptake aortic
rings were incubated with 0.118 to 11.8 µM ^{3}H-(-)NA for
2 min (MAO and COMT inhibited). The accumulated ^{3}H-radio-
activity was corrected for the amount of NA distributed
a) into the extracellular space (determined with ^{14}C-sor-
bitol) and b) into the extraneuronal (cocaine-resistant)
system. K_m was 2.3 µM and V_{max} 0.5 $nmol \cdot g^{-1} \cdot min^{-1}$.

The extraneuronal O-methylation of NA was determined by
incubation of nerve-free aortic rings with 0.118 to 59.1
µM ^{3}H-(-)NA for 2, 5 and 10 min (MAO inhibited). Initial
rates of O-methylation of NA were calculated from the
amount of normetanephrine (NMN) found in tissue and medium. The kinetic constants for O-methylation were K_m 3.6 µM
and V_{max} 0.6 $nmol \cdot g^{-1} \cdot min^{-1}$. Corticosterone (87 µM), a
blocker of the extraneuronal uptake of NA, greatly reduced
the formation of NMN, but to a lesser extent the removal
(accumulation and O-methylation) of NA. Obviously, NA distributed into two extraneuronal compartments, a cortico-
sterone-sensitive and a corticosterone-resistant one. Only
the former was associated with a high COMT activity. The
extraneuronal formation of NMN was hardly influenced by
neuronal uptake of NA, even at very low concentrations of
the amine (intact aorta, MAO inhibited), and there was
little or no formation of O-methylated metabolites in the
neurone. - The results indicate: a) the extraneuronal O-
methylation is an important mechanism for the elimination
of NA in the rabbit aorta and b) the extraneuronal uptake
of NA is hardly influenced by the neuronal uptake system.

Supported by the Deutsche Forschungsgemeinschaft
Dept. of Pharmacol., Univ. of Würzburg, D-8700 Würzburg

198

DISSOCIATION CONSTANTS AND PARTITION COEFFICIENTS OF
SYMPATHOMIMETIC AMINES,THEIR PRECURSORS AND METABO-
LITES   H.Bönisch and F. Mack

The dissociation constants (pK_a values) and the apparent
partition coefficients (log D values) of naturally occurring sympathomimetic amines, their precursors, and their
O-methylated and deaminated metabolites were determined.
These values were also estimated for a series of synthetic
sympathomimetic amines. The dissociation constants were
determined by potentiometric titration; the apparent partition coefficients were obtained from the ratio of the
concentration of the compound in the lipid phase (n-octa-
nol) to the concentration of the unionized plus ionized
species of the compound in the aqueous phase (phosphate
buffer pH 7.4).
The log D values were dependent on the pK_a values of the
substance. Methoxyhydroxymandelic acid (VMA), the acid
metabolite of noradrenaline and adrenaline, exhibited a
very low pK_a value and also a very low log D value, whereas
methoxyhydroxyphenylglycol (MOPEG) had   very high values
for both pK_a and log D. The apparent partition coefficients
of the metabolites of noradrenaline showed the following
ranking order: MOPEG>dihydroxyphenylglycol (DOPEG)> normetanephrine (NMN)>dihydroxymandelic acid (DOMA)> VMA.
The log D values were significantly correlated with the
rate constants for efflux of the metabolites of noradrenaline from the rat heart (reported by Fiebig and Trendelen-
burg: Naunyn-Schmiedeberg's Arch. Pharmacol. 293, Suppl.,R4,
1976). Based on the pK_a values of the compounds the log D
values were corrected to obtain log P values (pH independent partition coefficients). The substituent constants
(π values) of different substituents in the aromatic ring
and/or in the side chain of phenylethylamine were determined from the log P values.   (Supported by the DFG)

Institut für Pharmakologie und Toxikologie der Universität
D 87 Würzburg, Versbacher Landstrasse 9

199

UPTAKE OF 14-C-SEROTONIN BY HUMAN PLATELETS :
INFLUENCE OF THE TIME INTERVAL AFTER VENEPUNC-
TURE AND OF THE STORAGE TEMPERATURE
B. Lemmer and U. Jarosch

Human blood platelets are widely used as a neuronal model to study the effects of drugs on
the uptake of biogenic amines. In the present
study it was investigated whether various storage temperatures (4°,22°,37°C) and various
storage times (10-130 min) of the platelet-rich-
plasma (PRP) are able to influence the active
uptake of 14-C-5-HT studied at 37°C thereafter
as described earlier (Lemmer, Eur.J.Pharmacol.
21, 183, 1973). Both variables significantly
modified the V_{max} of the 5-HT uptake, but there
was no correlation with storage temperatures,
storage times or the changes in the pH of the
PRP. However, the K_m-value remained constant
(0.5µM).
At the storage temperature of 22°C, which is
usually used in these kind of experiments, studies with a competitive (amphetamine) and a
non-competitive (amantadine) 5-HT uptake inhibitor showed that the inhibitor constant of amphetamine (8 µM) was not influenced by the storage time, while the K_i-value of amantadine increased with time. Also 5-HT uptake inhibition
by propranolol, which is a mixed-type inhibitor
(Lemmer et al., Arch.Pharmacol. 275,299,1972),
decreased with storage time.
Thus, when using human blood platelets as a model to study the relative pharmacological effects of drugs, standardization of the storage
temperature of the PRP and of the time interval
after blood sampling is necessary.

Zentrum der Pharmakologie, J.W.Goethe-Universi-
tät, Theodor-Stern-Kai 7, D-6000 Frankfurt/Main

200

INHIBITION OF DOPAMINE RELEASE FROM RABBIT
NUCLEUS CAUDATUS BY APOMORPHINE AND BROMOCRIPTINE
W. Reimann, A. Zumstein and G. Hertting

Effects of dopamine receptor agonists and antagonists on the release of dopamine from rat
striatum have been studied repeatedly, but with
contradictory results (e.g., Farnebo and Hamberger, Acta physiol. scand. Suppl. 371, 35, 1971;
Dismukes and Mulder, Arch. Pharmacol. 297, 23,
1977). The following experiments were carried out
on frontally cut slices of the caudate nucleus of
the rabbit. The slices were preincubated with ^{3}H-
dopamine and then superfused with fresh medium
and stimulated by an electrical field at 3 Hz
(pulse duration 2 msec, 24 mA, stimulation
periods of 2 min).

The stimulation-evoked overflow of tritium was
calcium-dependent and tetrodotoxin-sensitive. It
was strongly reduced by apomorphine (0.01 - 1
µM). At 1 µM apomorphine, the inhibition amounted
to 77%. Bromocriptine (0.01-1 µM) also caused a
decrease. The effect of the agonists was antagonized by chlorpromazine (0.1 and 1 µM). Given
alone, chlorpromazine slightly augmented the
evoked overflow of tritium. The basal outflow
was not changed by the low concentrations indicated above, although it was accelerated by 10
µM of chlorpromazine as well as of apomorphine
and bromocriptine.

The results agree with the findings of Farnebo
and Hamberger (1971) on rat striatal slices.
They are compatible with the view that, in the
rabbit, a presynaptic dopaminergic negative
feedback mechanism controls the release of dopamine from nigro-striatal neurones.

Pharmakologisches Institut, Hermann-Herder-
Strasse 5, D-7800 Freiburg i.Br.

201

EFFECTS OF HALOTHANE ON THE NORADRENERGIC NEURONS OF THE RAT BRAIN CORTEX   M. Göthert

Administration of drugs which alter the noradrenaline concentration in the brain has been shown to modify the halothane concentration that is necessary for the induction of anaesthesia, suggesting that anaesthetics may affect noradrenergic pathways in the central nervous system (R.D. Miller, W.L. Way and E.I.Eger, II, Anesthesiology 29, 1153, 1968). To obtain more direct evidence for the ability of halothane to modify the function of central noradrenergic neurons, experiments were done in slices of the rat brain cortex. During incubation of the slices with (-)-3H-noradrenaline, halothane, decreased the accumulation of tritium. In slices preincubated with (-)-3H-noradrenaline, halo - thane accelerated the spontaneous efflux of tritium and inhibited the outflow induced by electrical field stimulation. The threshold concentration at which these effects were statistically significant varied between 0.28 and 0.95 mM. When the reuptake of (-)-3H-noradrenaline was blocked by 1 μM nomifensine, halothane caused a more pronounced inhibition of electrically stimulated tritium overflow.
It is concluded, that halothane is capable of inhibiting the impulse-induced noradrenaline release from noradrenergic neurons of the brain cortex.

Department of Pharmacology, University of Hamburg, Martinistr. 52, D-2000 Hamburg 20

202

IS HISTAMINE INVOLVED IN THE SYMPATHOMIMETIC EFFECT OF NICOTINE?   K. Starke

It has been proposed that histamine (HI) mediates the sympathomimetic effect of nicotine (NI) in the rabbit pulmonary artery (Chiou et al., Neuropharmacol. 15, 689, 1976). The hypothesis was examined on superfused artery strips. NI, HI and noradrenaline (NA) usually were applied at test concentrations of 30 μM (approximate EC_{50}), 30 μM (EC_{30}) and 0.1 μM (EC_{30}), respectively.

1) Pretreatment with 6-hydroxydopamine depleted the tissue of NA but not HI; the contractile effect of HI was unchanged, that of NA enhanced, that of NI abolished. 2) 0.01 μM (+)-chlorpheniramine reduced the response to HI. 10 μM was required to diminish the response to NI. At 10 μM, (-)-chlorpheniramine, which is a weaker antihistaminic drug than the (+)-enantiomer, also reduced the effect of NI. 3) 0.5 μM phenoxybenzamine irreversibly antagonized all three agonists. Receptor protection by 3000 μM HI preserved the effect of HI, but not NA and NI. Protection by 600 μM NA preserved the effect of both NA and NI, but not of HI. 4) Continuous exposure to 3000 μM HI produced a rapidly fading contraction. The artery was then refractory to HI, but normally sensitive to NA and NI. 5) After preincubation with 3H-NA, NI evoked an "explosive" tritium overflow. In contrast, HI caused a slowly developing increase in outflow. 6) The major part of the tritium overflow evoked by NI was 3H-NA. The outflow caused by HI almost entirely consisted of 3H-dihydroxyphenylglycol.

The results argue against a role of HI in the effect of NI. They support the view that NI acts by releasing NA via nicotine receptors on sympathetic nerve endings.

Pharmakologisches Institut, Hermann-Herder-Strasse 5, D-7800 Freiburg i. Br.

203

α-ADRENERGIC RECEPTORS IN HUMAN PLATELETS
K.H. Jakobs and R. Rauschek

Stimulation of human platelets by adrenaline and noradrenaline causes platelet aggregation and inhibition of platelet adenylate cyclase; both effects involve α-adrenergic receptors, since both are blocked by α-adrenergic blocking agents. The binding of [3H]dihydroergonine (3H-DHE), a potent α-adrenergic antagonist in the platelet system, was used to characterize the α-adrenergic receptors in both particulate preparations from human platelets and in intact platelets. Binding of 3H-DHE to platelet particles was rapid and reversible, with an association rate constant of $2.2 \cdot 10^7$ liters·mol^{-1}·min^{-1} and a dissociation rate constant of 0.027 min^{-1} at 25°. 3H-DHE binding was of high affinity, with an equilibrium dissociation constant (K_D) of 6.3 nM and was saturable with 220 fmol bound/mg of particle protein. No cooperativity was detectable. The α-adrenergic agonist (-)-adrenaline competed for 3H-DHE binding with a K_D of about 0.5 μM. The order of potencies for adrenergic agonists was (-)-adrenaline > (-)-noradrenaline (NA) ≫ (±)-methoxamine ≫ (-)-isoprenaline and for adrenergic antagonists was dihydroergonine > dihydroergotamine ≈ yohimbine > phentolamine ≫ tolazoline = azapetine ≫ (-)-propranolol = (-)-pindolol. (+)-NA was about 20 times less potent than (-)-NA. The specificities of the various agonists and antagonists for competition of 3H-DHE binding were in good agreement with their effects on platelet aggregation and adenylate cyclase. In intact platelets, binding of 3H-DHE reached equilibrium within about 10 min at 25° and was saturable with about 2000 binding sites/platelet.

Pharmakologisches Institut, Universität Heidelberg, Im Neuenheimer Feld 366, D-6900 Heidelberg

204

EFFECT OF A NEW ANTIHYPERTENSIVE DRUG, URAPIDIL, ON PRE- AND POSTSYNAPTIC α-ADRENOCEPTORS IN GUINEA-PIG AND RAT VAS DEFERENS   M. Eltze

Urapidil, phentolamine (both 10^{-8}-10^{-5}M), and clonidine (10^{-6}-10^{-5}M) competitively antagonized the effect of noradrenaline on postsynaptic α-adrenoceptors in organ bath-suspended rat vas deferens, yielding pA$_2$ values of 7.02, 7.64 and 5.81, respectively.
Affinity of clonidine (10^{-11}-10^{-5}M) and BAY 1470 (10^{-9}-10^{-5}M) to presynaptic α-adrenoceptors was calculated from dose response curves of these compounds to inhibit the twitch contractions of superfused vas deferens-hypogastric nerve preparation of the guinea-pig in response to nerve stimulation (pD$_2$=7.30 and 7.34, respectively). At high doses (10^{-6}-10^{-5}M), clonidine maximally produced 60% inhibition of the twitch hight, which appeared to be due to simultaneous α-blockade. Phentolamine (10^{-9}-10^{-4}M) had no effect on the preparation. At 10^{-11}-10^{-9}M, the urapidil dose-response curve parallels that of clonidine, from 10^{-8}-10^{-5}M the curve shifts to the right, compared with clonidine, generating only 36% maximal inhibition of twitch response, which suggests a simultaneous antagonism on α-receptors exerted by urapidil. Inhibition of twitches caused by submaximal concentrations of clonidine, BAY 1470, and urapidil was reversed by phentolamine, while urapidil failed to antagonize the inhibitory effects of clonidine and BAY 1470, respectively.
At lower concentrations, urapidil was observed to stimulate presynaptic α-adrenoceptors similar to clonidine and at higher doses to elicit α-blocking potency 4.2-fold weaker than phentolamine. These results indicate that in respect to pre- and postsynaptic α-adrenoceptors the action of this drug is complex but suggests a primary presynaptic stimulatory site of action not unrelated to α-adrenoceptor blockade.

Byk Gulden Lomberg Chemische Fabrik GmbH, Forschungslaboratorien, Byk-Gulden-Str. 2, D-7750 Konstanz

205

BLOCKING PROPERTIES OF 2-HALOGENO-3',4'-DIHYDROXY-ACETOPHENONE DERIVATIVES ON THE ALPHA-ADRENERGIC RECEPTOR. W. Christ, J. Schuster, R. Tertel, K. Quiring

In a previous communication, we have presented experimental data on several substratelike and productlike irreversible inhibitors of catechol-O-methyltransferase (Becker, Christ et al., Arch. Pharmacol., Suppl. II to 297, R 11, 1977): Molecules which are structural analogues of catecholamines and possess a highly reactive group were synthesized for example 2-chloro-3',4'-dihydroxyacetophenone (1), the corresponding 2-bromo derivative (2), 2-bromo-3',4'-dihydroxy-2-methylpropiophenone (3) and 2-chloro-4'-hydroxy-3'-methoxyacetophenone (4). Huidobro-Toro and Carpi have reported that compound 1 is a selective blocker of the α-adrenergic receptor (Arch. int. Pharmacodyn. 222, 180, 1976). It seemed of interest therefore, to see whether the α-adrenergic blocking properties of the molecule would change when chlorine would be replaced by bromine. In the "pithed" rat, the effects of the compounds 1-4 on the arterial hypertensive response to noradrenaline (NA) were tested. NA doses ranged from 0.1 µg/kg to 1 µg/kg. The effect of the alkylating reagents was investigated from 10 min to 120 min after application. Phenoxybenzamine (46 µg/kg) was used as reference substance. Compounds 1 and 4 produced adrenergic blockade during the time of observation in doses > 10 mg/kg to 32 mg/kg i.v.. These effects are comparable to those produced by phenoxybenzamine, but much higher doses were needed. The brominated compounds seem to be less effective as adrenergic blockers; this is tentatively attributed to their nonspecific binding to tissue proteins.

Institut für Arzneimittel, Bundesgesundheitsamt, Werner-Voß-Damm 62, D-1000 Berlin 42

206

FURTHER EVIDENCE FOR A SELECTIVE POST-SYNAPTIC α-ADRENOCEPTOR BLOCKADE WITH PRAZOSIN IN VASCULAR SMOOTH MUSCLE D. Cambridge, M. J. Davey and R. Massingham

Evidence to date indicates that pre- and post-synaptic α-adrenoceptors differ with respect to their affinities for both agonist (Starke, Endo and Taube, 1975) and antagonist drugs (Dubocovich and Langer, 1974; Starke, Borowski and Endo, 1975). Recently we have reported that prazosin has a marked affinity for post- as opposed to pre-synaptic α-adrenoceptors in the rabbit pulmonary artery (Cambridge, Davey and Massingham, 1977). Further experiments have been carried out to examine whether any interaction occurs between prazosin and an agonist and antagonist known to be selective for pre-synaptic α-adrenoceptors in rabbit pulmonary arteries. Interaction studies demonstrated that yohimbine caused a concentration dependent shift in the dose-response curve to clonidine at pre-synaptic α-adrenoceptors, but had little effect on the contractile activity of clonidine at post-synaptic α-adrenoceptors. By contrast, prazosin had little effect on the action of clonidine at pre-synaptic α-adrenoceptors, but caused a concentration dependent shift in the dose-response curve to clonidine at post-synaptic α-adrenoceptors. These observations demonstrate that prazosin, unlike yohimbine, has only affinity for post-synaptic α-adrenoceptors. In support of this conclusion it was found that prazosin, at concentrations sufficient to block the stimulation of post-synaptic α-adrenoceptors did not modify the action of yohimbine in promoting ^{3}HNA release via pre-synaptic α-adrenoceptor blockade. These results therefore provide further evidence that prazosin is a potent selective antagonist at the post-synaptic α-adrenoceptors in vascular smooth muscle which preserves the integrity of the pre-synaptically mediated negative feedback loop.

Department of Medicinal Biology, Biological Research Group, Pfizer Central Research, Sandwich, Kent, England.

207

β-ADRENOCEPTORS AND ADENYLCYCLASE ACTIVITY IN ERYTHROCYTES FROM RATS PRETREATED WITH ISOPRENALINE
G. Wiemer, D. Palm, G. Kremer, M. Reinhard

Specific desensitization of adrenergic receptors has been reported by several investigators (c.f. Wolfe et al. Ann.Pharmacol.Toxicol. 17, 575, 1977). It has been, therefore, investigated, whether adrenergic β-receptors in immature red blood cells from rats (after pretreatment with acetylphenylhydrazine 3x40 mg/kg) could be desensitized by treatment of the animals with high doses of ($\pm$) isoprenaline (Ipn; 4x30 mg/kg within 24 hours before decapitation). cAMP synthesis was measured in suspensions of intact cells or in membrane preparations; receptor density was determined using ^{3}H (-)-dihydroalprenolol (DHAP).

In intact cells from Ipn-treated animals cAMP-synthesis (basal and Ipn-stimulated) is strongly reduced by more than 50%. Also in membrane preparations basal as well as the Ipn stimulated adenylcyclase activity are decreased by > 50% without any change of the K_a-value. NaF (10^{-2}M) and GppNHp (10^{-4}M) stimulated enzyme activities, however, are decreased only by 30%. In vivo treatment with Ipn also lowers the B_{max}-values for DHAP - binding in membrane preparations (~20%) without any change of the respective K_D-value (8×10^{-9}M). Thus, treatment with Ipn elicits not only a reduction of the number of β-receptor sites but lowers also the concentration of adenylcyclase in immature red blood cells. The enzymatic unit appears to be more sensitive against the effects of high concentrations of catecholamines than the receptor unit.

Zentrum der Pharmakologie, J.W.Goethe-Universität, Th.-Stern-Kai 7, D-6000 Frankfurt/Main, FRG

208

CLASSIFICATION OF BETA-ADRENOCEPTOR SUB-TYPE MEDIATING RENIN RELEASE FROM THE JUXTAGLOMERULAR APPARATUS OF THE RAT G. Haeusler

Isolated rat kidneys were perfused through the renal artery with Krebs solution and the renin released in response to beta-adrenoceptor stimulants was measured in the venous effluent. Renin was determined with a radioimmunoassay for angiotensin I. Similarly, isolated rat hearts were perfused according to the technique of Langendorff and the increase in myocardial contractility in response to beta-adrenoceptor stimulants was measured with the use of a water-filled rubber balloon introduced into the left ventricle through the left atrium. Both for the kidney and the heart full dose-response curves of the non-selective isoprenaline and of terbutaline and salbutamol - two beta-adrenoceptor stimulants with relative specificity for the beta-2 sub-type - were constructed. The following respective EC_{50} values were found: 2.4×10^{-9}M, 3.4×10^{-6}M and 5.5×10^{-7}M (renin release) and 7.5×10^{-9}M, 3.4×10^{-6}M and 2.2×10^{-6}M (positive inotropic action). Arunlakshana and Schild plots indicated a competitive antagonism between isoprenaline and the non-selective beta-adrenoceptor blocking agents propranolol and bufuralol or the beta-1 selective blocking agent practolol with respective pA_{10} values of 1.4×10^{-8}M, 2.5×10^{-8}M and 1.3×10^{-6}M (kidney) and 1.6×10^{-8}M, 2.8×10^{-8}M and 2×10^{-6}M (heart). The beta-2 specific adrenoceptor blocking agent butoxamine did not antagonize the effect of isoprenaline in either preparation up to 10^{-6}M and produced an erratic antagonism with 10^{-5}M. It is concluded that cardiac and renal beta-adrenoceptors of the rat show a similar affinity for both agonists and antagonists with varying beta-1 or beta-2 selectivity and that on this basis the latter are classified as beta-1.

Pharma Research Department, F.Hoffmann-La Roche & Co.,Ltd., CH-4002 Basle, Switzerland

209

THE AFFINITY OF CARAZOLOL FOR MYOCARDIAL AND TRACHEAL
ß-ADRENOCEPTORS ACTIVATED BY (-)-ISOPRENALINE.
H.LEMOINE and A.J.KAUMANN

High affinity,tracheoselective ß-adrenoceptor antagonists
may be useful as tools to characterize smooth muscle
ß-adrenoceptors. We show that ($\pm$)-carazolol is a high
affinity, tracheoselective ligand.
In spontaneously beating right atria (RA) of kitten and
rat and in driven left atria (LA) (0.2 Hz) but not in
driven papillary muscles (PM) (0.5 Hz) of kitten,carazolol
caused positive chronotropic and inotropic effects (intrinsic activity of 0.1 with respect to isoprenaline (Iso) in
all tissues). The EC_{50} (-log M) for stimulation was 6.4 for
kitten RA, 7.2 for kitten LA and 6.5 for rat RA. In kitten
tissues the IC_{30} (-log M) was 4.5 for RA, 5.5 for LA and
5.3 for PM. The affinity of carazolol (B) was estimated
from its potency to antagonize the effects of Iso on RA,
LA, PM and trachea (relaxation of a carbachol induced contracture). 4 successive concentration-effect curves (CEC)
for Iso were determined on each tissue in the absence (control for spontaneous changes in sensitivity) and the presence of carazolol. Carazolol caused nearly parallel and sur-
mountable rightward shifts of the CEC for Iso. Concentration ratios (CR) of Iso $\bar{c}$ & $\bar{s}$ carazolol (corrected for
desensitization) were estimated to calculate the apparent
equilibrium dissociation constants $K_B = [B]/(CR-1)$. K_B's
(-log M) of carazolol were 10.0, 9.8 and 9.8 for kitten RA,
LA and PM, respectively, 9.9 and 11.4 for guinea pig RA
and trachea, resp., and 9.8 for rat RA. Mean slopes of
Schild plots for all groups (N$\geq$6/group) were 1.0 to 1.2.
Conclusions: 1)So far, carazolol is the ligand with highest
affinity for myocardial ß-adrenoceptors. 2)Carazolol has
30 times higher affinity for tracheal than for myocardial
ß-adrenoceptors. 3)Carazolol belongs to the class of non-
conventional partial agonists that only cause stimulation
at high ß-adrenoceptor occupancies (e.g. Pindolol).
(Supported in part by grant SFB 30 Kardiologie of the DFG).

Department of Clinical Physiology and Dep. of Pharmacology,
University of Düsseldorf, 4000 Düsseldorf, West Germany.

210

EFFECTS OF SOME DOPAMINE DERIVATIVES ON LIPID
AND CARBOHYDRATE METABOLISM. J. Puurunen* and
E. Westermann

It has been shown that xanthine derivatives of
dopamine are active in the cardiovascular system.
Compared with dopamine the derivatization produced a change of the pharmacological profile,
e.g. a shift in the activity and relative affinity for α- and β-adrenergic receptors (Anttila
et al. Naunyn-Schmiedeberg's Arch. Pharmacol.
297, Suppl. II, R 32, 1977).
In the present paper we investigated the lipolytic and glycogenolytic effects of some xanthine
derivatives of dopamine. In unanaesthetised rats
the i.m. injection of the 7-propyltheophylline
derivative of dopamine as well as its 7-(2-methyl)
-propyltheophylline and 7-(3-methyl)-propyl-
theophylline derivatives increased the plasma
level of free fatty acids and glycerol at 10-
100-times lower doses than dopamine. The maximal
effect of these derivatives on the plasma level
of glycerol was significantly greater and their
duration of action longer than those of dopamine.
The lipolytic effect of dopamine and its xanthine derivatives was antagonised by propranolol
(10 mg/kg i.m.). The plasma level of glucose was
elevated by the 7-(2-methyl)- and 7-(3-methyl)-
propyltheophylline derivatives at approx. 10-
times lower doses than by dopamine, but the maximal effect was - in contrast to lipolysis - not
greater than that of dopamine, indicating that
the glycogenolytic action of dopamine was less
affected by the derivatization.

Institut für Pharmakologie, Medizinische Hoch-
schule Hannover, Karl-Wiechert-Allee 9, 3000
Hannover 61
* Fellow of the Alexander von Humboldt Foundation
West Germany

211

BLOOD FLOW AND REGIONAL SYMPATHETIC ACTIVITY IN
THE SUPERIOR MESENTERIC VASCULAR BED DURING IN-
JECTION AND CONTINUOUS INFUSION OF DOPAMINE
R. Kullmann, R. Huß, K. Waßermann and R. Rissing

In 8 cats, anesthetized with chloralose-urethane,
dopamine was injected (25 µg/kg) and continuously
infused (5, 10, and 25 µg/kg min) into a femoral
vein or into the superior mesenteric artery. We
consecutively recorded superior mesenteric blood
flow and regional pre- and postganglionic sympathetic activity.
In response to the i.v. and i.a. bolus injections,
blood flow to the superior mesenteric vascular bed
increased by 53.7±35.5 % and by 59.9±49.2 % (mean
±S.D.; p=0.01). This vasodilation did not involve
significant changes in blood pressure and sympathetic activity. An initial vasoconstriction and
a concomitant rise in arterial mean blood pressure
consistently preceeded the vasodilation. During
this period pre- and postganglionic sympathetic
discharges were inhibited.
Continuous i.v. and i.a. infusion of dopamine elicited a dose dependent flow increase of 120.1±
83.2 % and 137.1±48.0 % at the highest dose (p=
0.01), which was regularly accompanied by a small
pressure drop (8.4±9.9 % and 7.3±5.4 %; p=0.05)
and by a slight increase in sympathetic activity,
significant changes being noted only for postganglionic discharges during intravenous infusion of
the drug.
These results provide evidence against the view
that mesenteric vasodilation evoked by therapeutic
doses of dopamine is mediated by an inhibition of
sympathetic mass discharges at ganglionic or preganglionic level.

Supported by the DFG

Pharmakologisches Institut der Universität Bonn,
Reuterstraße 2 b, D-5300 Bonn

212

THE INFLUENCE OF RESERPINE AND ADRENALECTOMY ON PLASMA CA-
TECHOLAMINE LEVELS AFTER ELEVATION OF INTRACRANIAL PRES-
SURE IN THE RAT AND IN THE CAT
N.Th.P. Roozekrans

Acute increase of intracranial pressure (ICP) in the anesthetized rat and cat caused a steep rise in arterial blood
pressure and different types of cardiac arrhythmia. This
cardiovascular response is apparently mediated by an increase in sympathetic activity and, therefore, we determined the arterial plasma levels of adrenaline (A) and of
noradrenaline (NA) during intracranial hypertension. ICP
was rapidly elevated to 160 mm Hg by introducing saline
under controlled pressure into the left lateral ventricle.
A-levels were measured by a fluorimetric method (Anton and
Sayre, J.Pharmacol. 138, 360, 1962), while NA-levels were
determined by a radioenzymatic technique (Henry et al.,
Life Scs. 16, 375, 1975). We investigated the influence of
reserpine on catecholamine levels in control animals and
bilaterally adrenalectomized cats and rats after increased
ICP. In the control rats the increase of ICP resulted in a
slow rise of catecholamine values, while the arterial blood
pressure rose immediately to a high level. NA-plasma concentrations achieved a maximum 10 minutes after onset of
cerebral hypertension, while A-concentrations reached a
maximal plateau after about 5 minutes. Intracranial hypertension in the control cat caused also a slow rise of NA-
levels with a maximum after 20 minutes, while no changes
in A-concentrations were observed. Blood pressure increased immediately after ICP-elevation. Bilateral adrenalectomy or pretreatment with reserpine diminished the increments of the NA-concentration after elevation of ICP. The
combination of both pretreatments did not influence the
plasma NA-level during increased ICP. Both pretreatment
with reserpine and bilateral adrenalectomy abolished the
rise in plasma A, in cats as well as in rats. We also determined the catecholamine concentrations in blood obtained
directly from a cannulated suprarenal vein.
Department of Pharmacy, Division of Pharmacotherapy,
University of Amsterdam,
Plantage Muidergracht 24, Amsterdam, The Netherlands.

213

ABOUT THE INFLUENCE OF ADENINE NUCLEOTIDES UPON THE RESPONSE OF VASCULAR SMOOTH MUSCLE TO ADRENERGIC DRUGS   W.Felix, G.Ringsgwandl

Experiments were performed on the perfused hindlimb of the cat (chloralose anesthesia) with registration of blood pressure, perfusion pressure, puls rate and venous volume of the perfused extremity concerning the vascular effects of adenosine (AD), norepinephrine (NE), Suprifen[R] (S), and isoprenaline (IP). After disappearance of the AD-induced (i.a.) dilatation a persisting increase of the α-adrenergic effects of NE and S was observed while the β-effect of IP was inhibited. After an infusion of AD following the i.a. application of NE or S there was a persistent rise in perfusion pressure above initial values. This increased α'-adrenergic effect was confirmed by experiments on rat aortic and portal vein strips: Following the application of AD (10^{-7} M) or ATP (10^{-7} M) a solution of 10^{-9} M NE or S caused a contraction as strong as NE or S (10^{-6} M) prior to the presence of AD (10^{-7} M) or ATP. This increase in contraction persisted also after elimination of AD or ATP from the organ bath and was reversibly blocked by dipyridamole or Mg^{++}. This increased NE- and S-contraction was only present when NE was given at the beginning of the experiment. The reproducibility of our results was not been satisfactory until now as the effect described was seen in about 80 of 110 animals only.

University Department of Pharmacology
Nußbaumstr.26, D-8000 München 2

214

BIOISOSTERISM IN THE FIELD OF PARASYMPATHOMIMETICS   G. Lambrecht

If a molecularly modified drug is to react at the same sites as the original drug to bring about the desired action, the molecular modification should not be too drastic. It can be rationalized by substituting one atom or group of atoms in the parent compound for another with a similar electronic and steric configuration. In the course of earlier studies with cyclic acetylcholine analogues in the saturated 6-membered ring series, it was found, that the replacement of the ammonium group in piperidine analogues by the sulfonium group is accompanied by a dramatic increase of the muscarinic potency(G.Lambrecht, Eur.J.Med.Chem.12,41(1977)). The present work describes investigations with compounds in the acetyl-gamma-homocholine series: 1-methyl and 1,1-dimethyl-4-acetoxypiperidine(1 and 2), cis- and trans-4-acetoxy-1-methylthianium(3 and 4). 1 - 4 interact with the muscarinic receptor directly and specifically. The stereochemistry was investigated with NMR, MO calculations and X-Ray. Kinetic data obtained were used to characterize the biological activity.

MUSCARINIC ACTIVITY(g.-p. atrium, contraction)

	ED_{50} (M)	K (M x 10^8)	$t_{1/2}$ (sec, ED_{50})
Ach	3.85×10^{-8}	2.36	19.1
1	7.01×10^{-6}	568	30.8
2	7.40×10^{-6}	850	23.8
3	2.10×10^{-8}	2.57	16.5
4	1.91×10^{-6}	194	14.2

Department of Pharmacology, University of Frankfurt, D 6000 Frankfurt, Robert-Mayer-Strasse 7/9

215

IN VITRO AND IN VIVO BINDING STUDIES ON THE INTERACTIONS OF PSYCHOTROPICS DRUGS WITH MUSCARINIC RECEPTORS J.Laszlo, H. Bittiger, and L. Maître.

A combination of in vitro and in vivo ^{3}H-quinuclidinyl-benzylate (QNB) radioreceptor assays (Yamamura et al., PNAS 71, 1725, 1974; Brain. Res. 80, 170, 1974) was used to study the anticholinergic properties of various antidepressants and neuroleptics. In vitro, inhibition of ^{3}H-QNB (1nM) binding by psychotropic drugs was determined on rat cortex membranes. In vivo, ^{3}H-QNB was injected intravenously (7,5 nmoles/rat) 30 or 60 min after atropine or the psychotropics. Brains were removed 1 h later. Accumulation of radioactivity was determined in various brain regions. The anticholinergic effects of atropine, classical antidepressants and neuroleptics in the rat cortex under these conditions are given in the Table. The inhibitions were concentration or dose-dependent. After treatment with increasing doses of the psychotropics a plateau was reached at approximately 50% inhibition. Analyses of the data showed that both the in vitro and the in vivo tests are necessary to predict the presence of potential anticholinergic side effects of psychotropics agents.

Drug	In vitro (IC_{50},nM)	In vivo (ED_{20},mg/kg,i.p.)
Atropine	5	1.5
Clozapine	100	0.3
Chlorpromazine	2000	> 30
Imipramine	700	10
Amitriptyline	70	3

* Values refer to 20 % inhibition of ^{3}H-QNB Binding.

Research Department, Pharmaceuticals Division,
CIBA-GEIGY Ltd., Basle, Switzerland.

216

DETERMINATION OF THE SUBCELLULAR ORIGIN OF [14C] ACETYLCHOLINE (ACh) AND [3H] ACETYLPYRROLIDINECHOLINE (APyCh) RELEASED FROM GUINEA-PIG CEREBRAL CORTEX AFTER ELECTRICAL STIMULATION I. von Schwarzenfeld

After in vivo application of radiolabelled choline, radioactive ACh is formed and can be released from the brain by electrical stimulation. However, its origin is still obscure because, due to the metabolical heterogeneity of synaptic vesicles, no subcellular compartment has been found with a specific activity (SA) corresponding to that of released transmitter. To bypass this heterogeneity problem, two different labelled precursors can be used.

Cups filled with Locke's solution containing paraoxon (100 µM) were placed on guinea-pig cerebral cortex. [3H] pyrrolidinecholine (72 µCi) and [14C] choline (12 µCi) were injected into the cortical tissue underneath the cup (1.5 mm depth). Uptake of transmitter into the vesicles was enhanced by low frequency electrical stimulation (0.1 Hz) of this area and release (approx. doubling spontaneous release) provoked by high frequency stimulation (30 Hz). Cortex underlying the cup was removed, fractionated and radioactive transmitters extracted from the cytoplasm (0), the vesicle fraction (D) and a fraction containing presynaptic membranes with vesicles attached (H).

In unstimulated controls, the molar ratio [14C] ACh/[3H] APyCh in the cup solution was found to be similar to that in the cytoplasm (cup=31.3 + 1.0; 0=27.3 + 2.2; H=18.1 + 2.2; n=3). However, after stimulation it approximated to that in fraction H (cup = 17.2 + 2.0; H=18.1 + 0.8; 0= 31.0 + 1.6; n=5). We conclude that the transmitter released from guinea-pig cortex after electrical stimulation might origin mainly from a small, metabolically very active vesicular pool closely attached to the presynaptic membrane.

Pharmakologisches Institut der Universität Mainz,
Obere Zahlbacher Str. 67, D-6500 Mainz

217

EFFECTS OF ATROPINE ON ACETYLCHOLINE OVERFLOW FROM PER-FUSED CHICKEN HEARTS   H. Kilbinger and C. Krieg

Isolated chicken hearts were perfused (20 ml/min) with Tyrode's solution. Release of acetylcholine (ACh) was evoked either by electrical stimulation (1 ms; 15 mA) of both preganglionic vagus nerves or by perfusion with dimethylphenylpiperazinium (DMPP). ACh was extracted from the perfusates by ion-pair extraction and determined by gas chromatography.

Atropine (1 µM in all experiments) did not modify the ACh overflow caused by stimulation at 3 Hz (255 $\pm$ 55 pmol/g x 2 min; N = 4), but slightly increased the overflow at 20 Hz (from 465 $\pm$ 62 to 672 $\pm$ 82 pmol/g x 2 min; N = 5; p < 0.05). When the hearts were perfused with an eserine (1 µM) containing Tyrode's solution the ACh output at 3 Hz (457 $\pm$ 99 pmol/g x 2 min; N = 6) was not different from that caused by 20 Hz in the absence of cholinesterase inhibition. However, atropine in the presence of eserine led to a 4.1 fold increase of ACh overflow at 3 Hz.

The ACh overflow during a 2 min perfusion with 3×10^{-4} M DMPP either in the absence (163 $\pm$ 49 pmol/g; N = 4) or in the presence of 1 µM eserine (330 and 353 pmol/g; 2 expts.) was unaffected by atropine.

The experiments with DMPP support the idea (1) that the postganglionic parasympathetic nerve terminals of the chicken heart are not equipped with muscarine receptors that modulate ACh release. It is concluded that atropine increases the overflow of ACh evoked by preganglionic nerve stimulation by blocking inhibitory ganglionic muscarine receptors.

(1) Kilbinger, H., E. Hilgert: Meeting of German and Italian Pharmacologists, Venezia 1977, Abstract p. 371

Pharmakologisches Institut der Universität Mainz, Obere Zahlbacher Str. 67, D-6500 Mainz

218

THE EFFECT OF ANTICHOLINERGICS ON FOUR PARAMETERS RECORDED SIMULTANEOUSLY IN RATS   H. Hummelt, H.M. Jennewein, and F. Waldeck

Pharmacological investigations on differentiated effects of anticholinergic drugs on the gastric or salivary secretion are generally carried out on various species (rat, mouse). In order to exclude any possible differences present in the species in these experiments, an experimental procedure was set up in which the influence on organ functions stimulated peripherially and cholinergically by anticholinergics can be investigated in one experimental animal (anaesthetized rat). In this case the gastric secretion is determined according to the method of Lai (Gut 5: 327,1964). At the same time the mouth cavity is perfused with physiological NaCl and the salivary secretion is recorded gravimetrically as the difference between the quantity entering into and flowing out of the mouth cavity. In addition the small intestinal motility is recorded with a balloon catheter as well as the heart rate with the ECG.
The subcutaneous administration of 0.025 mg/kg carbachol causes clear stimulation of gastric and salivary secretion, of small intestinal motility as well as a decrease of the heart rate. This shows that these 4 parameters can be recorded in one model.
The administration of 0.01 mg/kg i.v. atropin completely antagonised all carbachol effects. In contrast to this only the effects on salivary secretion and heart rate were abolished by α,α-diphenyl-γ-piperidyl-butyramide HCl (Hoe-9980, 0.01 mg/kg i.v.). On the other hand only the effects on gastric secretion and the heart rate are antagonised by (-)N-ethyl-norscopolamin-methobromide (Ba-253, 0.001 mg/kg i.v.). These results show that a differentiated action between gastric and salivary secretion can occur with anticholinergic drugs.

C.H. Boehringer Sohn, D 6507 Ingelheim

219

EFFECTS OF OUABAIN AND ADENOSINE ON EXTRACELLULAR Ca^{2+} AND K^+, AS MEASURED WITH ION SELECTIVE MICROELECTRODES IN CEREBELLAR CORTEX
G. ten Bruggencate, R. Steinberg

Extracellular Ca^{2+} and K^+ levels ($|Ca^{2+}|_e$, $|K^+|_e$) were recorded with ion selective microelectrodes in the cerebellar cortex. Repetitive (10-20 Hz) stimulation of a parallel fiber beam evoked an increase in $|K^+|_e$ from its resting level (3 mmol/l) to about 8 mmol/l, whereas $|Ca^{2+}|_e$ decreased from 1.2 to about 0.9 mmol/l.

Ouabain and K-strophantidin (10^{-5}-$5 \cdot 10^{-5}$ mol/l) applied in the superfusion solution (n=9) caused a rise in $|K^+|_e$ from 3.19 $\pm$ 0.15 to 6.15 $\pm$ 1.79 mmol/l, paralleled by a Ca^{2+}-decrease from 1.12 $\pm$ 0.09 to 0.62 $\pm$ 0.16 mmol/l. K^+-transients evoked by repetitive stimulation were diminished, their decay phases prolonged and undershoots reduced.

Adenosine ($5 \cdot 10^{-3}$ mol/l) and Cl-adenosine ($5 \cdot 10^{-4}$ mol/l) diminished the amplitude of the stimulation-induced Ca^{2+}-decrease and K^+-increase. Mn^{2+} ($2 \cdot 10^{-3}$ mmol/l) had similar, although stronger, actions, i. e. it abolished stimulus-evoked Ca^{2+}-signals and reduced (secondarily) K^+-signals.

The results suggest 1) that the extracellular Ca^{2+}-level in the CNS is dependent on active transport processes, which in turn can be blocked by glycosides, and 2) that adenosine may act as a Ca^{2+}-antagonist also in the CNS.

Department of Physiology, University of München, Pettenkoferstraße 12, D-8000 München 2

220

EFFECTS OF ANESTHETICS ON THE CELLULAR REGULATION OF ENERGY METABOLISM.
E.Hering, H.Höfeler, J.Krieglstein, and K.Wever
It has been demonstrated in previous work that hexokinase is solubilized from the mitochondrial membrane in anesthesia (Bielicki and Krieglstein, Naunyn-Schmiedeberg's Arch. Pharmacol. 289, 61 and 229, 1977).This effect was strongly correlated with the surgical stage of anesthesia but its significance for anesthesia is not clear. In the study presented we treated male Spraque-Dawley rats with the antimetabolite 6-aminonicotinamide (6-AN) in order to elevate the cerebral concentration of glucose 6-phosphate which is the most potent substrate for the solubilization of bound hexokinase. After intraperitoneal injection of 6-AN (35mg/kg) to rats 17 h before decapitation, we measured an increased activity of soluble brain hexokinase in the same order of magnitude as it was determined in anesthesia. However, the 6-AN treated rats did not show distinct signs of anesthesia.Therefore the possibility seems to be ruled out that the solubilization of hexokinase from the outer mitochondrial membrane might be the only cause for the anesthetic effect. The question arises whether other capabilities of the mitochondrial membrane are altered by anesthetics, too.A possible influence of the anesthetics on the adenine nucleotide carrier seems to be most interesting. Therefore we prepared rat liver mitochondria and examined this carrier according to Duée and Vignais (J. biol. Chem. 244, 3932, 1969). It was demonstrated that already a concentration of 10^{-5}M thiopental inhibits the adenine nucleotide translocation across the inner mitochondrial membrane.

Institut für Pharmakologie und Toxikologie im FB Pharmazie der Philipps-Universität, Ketzerbach 63, D-3550 Marburg

221

EFFECT OF HALOTHANE ON THE SURVIVAL TIME OF TETANUS
INTOXICATED MICE   S. Huck, G. Gogolák, R. Jindra
and Ch. Stumpf
_____

Local tetanus of the rabbit has been used as a method of
assessing the anti-tetanus potency of various drugs
(Laurence, D. R. and Webster, R. A., Brit. J. Pharmacol.
13, 1958, 330-333). For evaluating the activity of drugs
against experimental general tetanus a model is presented,
based on the estimation of the survival time of mice.

Male mice (Swiss albino, Chemie Linz A.G., 22 ± 1 g;
room temperature $25 \pm 1^{\circ}C$) were injected subcutaneously
with 500 LD_{50} tetanus toxin (Behringwerke, Marburg). Eight
to nine hours later the onset of convulsive fits could be
observed in the control group. The mice were exposed to
0.35 % v/v halothane seven hours after the application of
the toxin, until the mortality reached 70 %. Halothane was
used as antagonist, since this agent can be administered
to the animals in a constant concentration for several
hours. The results presented in the table show that in
comparison to the control group the duration of survival
is significantly increased under the influence of a sub-
anesthetic halothane concentration.

mortality %

	hours after the injection of the toxin								
9^{30}	10	10^{30}	11	11^{30}	12	12^{30}	13	13^{30}	14	14^{30}
C: 4	12	30	54	74	90	94	98	100	
H:	3	8	19	22	30	41	56	63	69	72

C: control (N = 50)   H: halothane (N = 90)

Our preliminary experiments with halothane suggest that
the estimation of the survival time of mice might be a
suitable method for sceening drugs for their anti-tetanus
potency.

Department of Neuropharmacology, University of Vienna and
Brain Research Inst., Austrian Academy of Sciences,
Währingerstr. 13 a, A 1090 Vienna, Austria

222

Antagonism of acute pyrazidol overdosage in the mouse
P.A. Martorana, U. Heucke and R.-E. Nitz
_____

Pyrazidol is a tetracyclic pyrazino-indole derivative
with antidepressant activity. Acute overdosage of
pyrazidol in laboratory animals was found to result in
clonic convulsions and death. A dose-response relationship (i.p.) for convulsive activity and lethality
was determined in mice. The two curves were parallel
and all animals which died showed convulsions prior to
death. To investigate an effect upon the pyrazidol-
induced toxicity various drugs were injected (i.p.)
30 minutes prior to a convulsive dose (90-100) or a
lethal dose (90-100) of pyrazidol. Diazepam (D) and
phenobarbital sodium (P) were effective both against
convulsions and lethality. However while D was active
at similar doses against convulsions and lethality P
was approximately five times less potent against convulsions than against lethality. Clonidine was partially
effective in both models, cyproheptadine was partially
effective against convulsions only and chlorpromazine,
diphenylhydantoine, propranolol and phenoxybenzamine
were inactive in both models. D and P were also
effective against lethality when injected ten minutes
after pyrazidol. In this regard D was effective at
similar doses as when injected prior to pyrazidol while
P was effective at doses approximately five time higher.

These results indicate that both D and P are effective
against pyrazidol overdosage, in this respect however
D was more potent and more specific.

Department of Medical Biological Research,
CASSELLA FARBWERKE MAINKUR AG, Hanauer Landstr. 526
6000 Frankfurt/Main 61, BRD

223

INTERACTIONS OF ANTICONVULSANTS AND NEUROLEPTICS IN EX-
PERIMENTAL SEIZURES   H.J. Teschendorf, W. Worstmann,
and R. Kretzschmar
_____

In general neuroleptics have no anticonvulsive properties
but in contrast induce or enhance seizures (T.M. Itil and
J.P. Meyers, in Anticonvulsant drugs, Vol. 2, p. 608,
Pergamon press, 1973). Experimental data on the interactions of anticonvulsants with neuroleptics has not yet
been found. Therefore we investigated in mice the effects
of orally given melperone (mel), haloperidol (hal), chlorpromazine (cpz), and thioridazine (thi) separately and
partially in combination with diphenylhydantoin (dph),
dipropylacetate (dpa), trimethadione (tri) or diazepam
(dia) using the min. and the max. electroshock seizure
test (MinES, MES) and the max. pentetrazol seizure test
(MPS). Only mel (a butyrophenone neuroleptic with sedative
and weak anticonvulsive properties (Christensen et al.,
Acta pharmacol. et toxicol., 23, 109, 1965) showed anticonvulsive effects in all 3 tests (ED 50: 84; 53; 107
mg/kg resp.). CPZ was only effective in the MinES (ED 50:
57 mg/kg). Hal and thi were ineffective in all tests. The
anticonvulsive action of dph was clearly diminished by all
the neuroleptics tested in MES,resp. by mel tested in MPS.
In contrast, the action of dia in MES and MPS was augmented. Combinations of mel with dia acted synergistic,
those with mel and tri or dpa nearly additive against
tonic seizures. The anticonvulsive action of dia, tri and
dpa on clonic convulsions (MinES) was mostly augmented by
the neuroleptics; antagonism was never found. The results
show, that in mice neuroleptics have a antagonistic influence only on the antitonic antiepileptic dph. The anticonvulsive action of the also anticlonic active drugs dia,
tri and dpa was either augmented by the neuroleptics or
not influenced.

Department für Pharmakologie, Sparte Pharma, BASF Aktien-
gesellschaft, 6700 Ludwigshafen (Rhein)

224

DISTRIBUTION OF VALPROATE ACROSS THE INTERFACE
BETWEEN BLOOD AND CEREBROSPINAL FLUID.
W. Löscher and H.-H. Frey
_____

The entry of valproate into the cerebrospinal
fluid (CSF) was studied in dogs anesthetized by
pentobarbital and relaxed by suxamethonium.
Steady state concentrations of the rather
strong acid (pK_a 4.56) in CSF were reached
within 1 h, they corresponded exactly to the
concentration of free drug in serum. Probenecid
considerably enhanced the rate of entry into
CSF, and the ratio between concentrations in CSF
and free valproate in serum rose to a value of
1.5. An increase in this ratio could also be
induced by a strong acidosis (pH 6.9-7.2 in
blood). Neither probenecid nor acidosis had an
influence on the binding of valproate to serum
proteins. Phenylbutazone displaced valproate
from its protein binding and gave rise to
higher concentrations in CSF, but the ratio of
valproate concentrations in CSF and free drug
in serum remained at 1.0. The results suggest
a transport of valproate into and out of CSF,
probably by the monocarboxylic acid system.
Diffusion should only play a minor role. (DFG)

Lab. of Pharmacology and Toxicology, School of
Veterinary Medicine, Free University Berlin,
Koserstr. 20, D-1000 Berlin-West 33

225

PHARMACOKINETICS OF ETHOSUXIMIDE IN THE DOG.
Mossad A. El Sayed

The pharmacokinetics of ethosuximide was studied in dogs after intravenous and oral administration. Ethosuximide was determined by gas chromatography. After iv. injection of 20, 40 or 60 mg/kg, a monophasic exponential decay of the serum concentration was found, suggesting the validity of a one compartment open model. The half-life of elimination was 18+ 4 h with a tendency to longer half-lives with the higher doses. The apparent volume of distribution amounted to about 67 % of body weight. Ethosuximide rapidly crossed the blood-brain barrier: steady-state concentrations in cerebrospinal fluid were reached within 30 min, they corresponded to the fraction not bound to serum proteins (98 %). After oral administration, the drug was readily and completely (90 %) absorbed, maximal serum concentrations were reached within 0.8 to 4 h. Serum concentrations during prolonged administration (3 daily doses for 5-8 days) were predictable on the basis of the pharmacokinetic data determined with single doses up to maximal serum concentrations of 120 mg/l. The pharmacokinetics of ethosuximide in the dog correspond better to the values known from man (half-life 50 h) than those in rats (half-life 10 h) or mice (half-life 1 h). (DFG)

Lab. of Pharmacology and Toxicology, School of Veterinary Medicine, Free University Berlin, Koserstr. 20, D-1000 Berlin-West 33

226

EFFECT OF SINGLE AND REPEATED TREATMENT WITH ANTIDEPRESSANTS ON CLONIDINE-INDUCED HYPOACTIVITY IN THE RAT
A. DELINI-STULA

Owing to its selective presynaptic α-receptor stimulating action, clonidine decreases the liberation of the NA into the synaptic cleft. In rats low doses of clonidine depress the motor activity and this is believed to be causally related to the diminished NA release. We have investigated the effect of single and repeated treatment with imipramine, maprotiline and mianserine on clonidine (0.1 mg/kg)-induced hypoactivity in the rat. Imipramine and maprotiline do not show any appreciable extent of pre-, but rather pronounced postsynaptic α-blocking action. Mianserine, in contrast, blocks also presynaptic α-receptors (Baumann, P.A. and L. Maitre, Naunyn-Schmiedeberg's Arch. Pharmacol. 300, 31, 1977). Single doses of imipramine and maprotiline (2.5-10 mg/kg i.p.) were found to potentiate clonidine-induced hypoactivity, but a tolerance to this effect developed after repeated (daily for 5 days) administration of these drugs. Mianserine (25 mg/kg i.p.) antagonized slightly but significantly clonidine-induced depression and this antagonism was rather increased after 5 days of treatment. The results indicate that functional state of postsynaptic α-receptors changes in the course of repeated treatment with antidepressants, probably in the sense of an increased reactivity to NA.

Research Department, Pharmaceuticals Division, CIBA-GEIGY Ltd., Basel, Switzerland.

227

SUBSTANCE P IN CIRCULATING BLOOD: ORIGIN AND ELIMINATION
F. Lembeck, R. Gamse, M. Schweditsch and P. Holzer

Substance P (SP) in plasma of fasted cats was found to be 69.3±9.8 fmol/ml (SEM, n = 25, radioimmunassay of extracted plasma). Evisceration lowered the concentration to 28.7±9.0 % (n = 5, p < 0.01) after 15 min and to 24.7±9.9 % (n = 4, p < 0.01) after 60 min. Ligation of all intestinal arteries and the portal vein reduced the concentration to 55.4±14.1 % (n = 7, p < 0.05). No difference between the concentration of SP in portal plasma and in plasma of the V. cava inferior was found (71.8±11.2 versus 68.3±12.1 fmol/ml, n = 6). These results suggest, that the origin of circulating SP is mainly the intestine.

Elimination of SP from the circulation was studied in the rat. SP (1 μg/5 min) was infused into different vascular beds and the salivary secretion used as bioassay. The range of elimination was: liver > hind leg >> kidney > lung > brain. Elimination by the perfused isolated rat hind quarter and inactivation by rat plasma was temperature dependent. Plasma half life of SP in vitro was 12 min at 37°. From these results it can be concluded that circulating SP is inactivated in plasma as well as in organs.

Institut für Experimentelle und Klinische Pharmakologie, Universitätsplatz 4, A-8010 G r a z

228

SUBSTANCE P AND SYNAPTIC VESICLES: CHARACTERISTICS OF BINDING
N. Mayer and A. Saria

The binding of substance P(SP) to synaptic vesicles from rat brain was studied by incubation of ^{125}J-Tyr-8-SP with synaptic vesicles at 30°C. The incubation was terminated by transfer of SP into an organic phase (petroleum ether: chloroform 2:1)(modified method of Lembeck et al., Naunyn Schmiedeberg's Arch. Pharmacol. 297 Suppl. II, R55(1977)). The binding of SP to synaptic vesicles was shown to be saturable, its K_D was 3.57×10^{-11}M. The number of binding sites was calculated as 0.81×10^{-12} Mol/mg Protein. Scatchard analysis showed only one population of binding sites. ^{125}J-Tyr-8-SP bound to synaptic vesicles under saturation conditions could be displaced by an excess of SP with rate constants $k_1 = 3.04 \times 10^5$ Mols^{-1} and $k_{-1} = 1.06 \times 10^{-3}$ Mols^{-1}. 10^{-4}M SP leads to a complete displacement of ^{125}J-Tyr-8-SP from vesicles. These results are in agreement with observations of Kitabgi et al. (Proc. Natl. Acad. Sci. 74, 1846-1850(1977)) obtained from Neurotensin binding to synaptic membranes. No degradation of SP during incubation was observed.
Conclusion:
The binding of SP to synaptic vesicles was found to be highly specific, saturable and reversible to only one population of binding sites. The existance of a receptor or storage site for SP in synaptic vesicles is in agreement with a role as neurotransmitter or -modulator.

Institut für Experimentelle und Klinische Pharmakologie Universitätsplatz 4, A-8010 G r a z

229

INHIBITION OF TAURINE UPTAKE INTO AND RELEASE FROM P$_2$-FRACTIONS PREPARED FROM KAINIC ACID LESIONED RAT CORPORA STRIATA.   P.Placheta and E.Singer

Stereotaxic injections of kainic acid (KA) into the corpus striatum lead to a destruction of striatal interneurons. Axons passing through or terminating in the area seem to be unaffected(Schwarcz, R.& Coyle,J.T.,Brain Res.127,235,1977).
Since taurine exhibits some neurotransmitter properties in the CNS and is present in the striatum in high concentrations, the effect of local KA-injections on the uptake and release of ^{3}H-taurine was studied in vitro using P$_2$-(crude synaptosomal) fractions. Experiments with ^{14}C-GABA and ^{3}H-dopamine (DA) were included to examine the extent and specificity of the lesions.
Adult rats received a unilateral injection of 2μg of KA into the striatum and were killed 10 days after lesion. Endogenous levels of taurine were reduced to about 73% and of GABA to 25% of the uninjected (control) side. Uptake of ^{3}H-taurine and ^{14}C-GABA into P$_2$-fractions prepared from the lesioned side was reduced to 78% and 37% of controls, respectively; ^{3}H-DA uptake was not significantly altered. In superfusion experiments with preloaded P$_2$-fractions K$^+$-(56mM)induced release of ^{3}H-taurine and ^{14}C-GABA was reduced to 63% and 41% of controls; ^{3}H-DA release remained unchanged.
These data suggest that in the striatum of the rat a considerable portion of taurine is localized in interneurons. In addition, the results present further evidence for a selective destruction of striatal gabaergic interneurons by local injection of KA without affecting dopaminergic nerve terminals.

Pharmakologisches Institut der Universität Wien, A-1090 Wien, Währingerstraße 13a

230

EFFECTS OF DIAZEPAM AND BACLOFEN ON THE GABA TURNOVER RATE IN VARIOUS MOUSE BRAIN REGIONS. R. Bernasconi and P. Martin

By blocking the GABA catabolism to succinic semialdehyde with the irreversible GABA-transaminase inhibitor gabaculine, the rate of GABA synthesis can be estimated from the initial linear increase in GABA concentration in mouse brain regions. Baclofen (0.3 mg/kg i.p. to 10 mg/kg i.p.) and diazepam (0.01 mg/kg to 10 mg/kg i.p.) did not change GABA steady state concentration. However, they both caused a dose-dependent reduction of the GABA turnover in the four brain regions studied, namely in the cerebellum, cerebral cortex, hippocampus and c. striatum. With baclofen the effect was stereospecific as the (+) isomer was inactive up to 10 mg/kg i.p. Muscimol, (1.5 mg/kg i.p.) a potent and specific GABA receptor agonist did not change GABA content in these regions but depressed GABA turnover rate.
The similarity of action of the three drugs on GABA rate of synthesis further supports the theory that diazepam and baclofen may act as GABA-mimetic drugs.

Research Department, Pharmaceuticals Division, CIBA-GEIGY Ltd., Basle, Switzerland.

231

EFFECT OF BACLOFEN APPLIED TO THE SUBSTANTIA NIGRA ON STRIATAL LEVELS OF DOPAMINE, 5-HT AND THEIR METABOLITES. P.C. Waldmeier, J.-J. Feldtrauer, R. Kam and K. Stöcklin
2.5 μg baclofen (B) in 1 μg saline were injected into the right s. nigra of rats with preset cannula guides and dopamine (DA), homovanillic (HVA), 3,4-dihydroxyphenylacetic (DOPAC), 5-hydroxyindoleacetic (5-HIAA) acids and serotonin (5-HT) measured in ipsi- and contralateral striata .5, 1, 2, 4, and 6 h after injection. 5 rats were in a group, and saline controls were used. On the injected side, DA levels rose to 165% of saline control after 30 min and 184 % after 2 h. The effect subsided thereafter, control levels being reached at 6 h. HVA decreased initially (50% after 1 h), then increased to 304% at 4 h. Normal levels were observed at 6 h. DOPAC was unchanged for the first h, then increased to a max. of 185% at 4 h. Normalization occurred after 6 h. 5-HT levels increased with a max. of 179% after 2 h and 5-HIAA with a max. of 144% after 4 h. 5-HT, but not 5-HIAA,was normal after 6 h. Contralaterally, DA was unchanged. HVA, DOPAC, 5-HT and 5-HIAA rose between 20 and 100%. Maxima varied between .5 and 2 h, and normalization occurred after 6 h. The ipsilateral rise in DA levels and the initial drop in HVA are interpreted as being due to inhibition of impulse flow in the DA neurons by B. The subsequent increases of HVA and DOPAC may be related to intraneuronal metabolism of excess DA. The contralateral rise of HVA and DOPAC may reflect a compensatory increase in impulse flow in these DA neurons. The effect of B on 5-HT and 5-HIAA was similar in time course to that after i.p. injection, though the increase in 5-HIAA was relatively smaller. A dose-response curve (.313 - 1.25 ug; 3 h) showed B effects on DA and 5-HT to occur at similar doses, as after i.p. injection. No significant effect on 5-HIAA was observed, however. B effects on striatal 5-HT, in contrast to those on 5-HIAA, may be related to the drug's effect on nigro-striatal DA-system.
Departement Forschung, Div. Pharma, CIBA-GEIGY AG, Basel.

232

THE ANTI-NOCICEPTIVE ACTION OF SUBSTANTIA NIGRA STIMULATION AND SOME OF ITS PHARMACOLOGICAL ASPECTS I.Jurna and G.Heinz
In rats with the brains either left intact or transected at the prenigral plane, repetitive stimulation of the substantia nigra prolonged the reaction time of the tail-flick, increased the reflex discharges from extensor α motoneurones and reduced the α reflex latency. Naloxone (1 mg/kg) failed to influence the anti-nociceptive effect of nigral stimulation but antagonized the facilitation of monosynaptic α reflex discharge. Morphine (2 mg/kg) did not alter the α reflex discharges without and during nigral stimulation, but shortened the reflex latency and abolished the antagonistic effect of naloxone on nigral conditioning. The anti-nociceptive effect of morphine observed in intact rats was abolished by prenigral decerebration and restored by additional spinalization. The results indicate that (1) the substantia nigra influences flexor (nociceptive) and extensor reflex activity in a reciprocal manner independent of an intact nigro-striatal feedback loop, and (2) morphine affects the nociceptive reflex by an action at different levels of the central nervous system.

Pharmakologisches Institut der Universität des Saarlandes, 665 Homburg/Saar, FRG

233

IN VIVO RELEASE OF ENDOGENOUS CATECHOLAMINES AND GABA IN THE HYPOTHALAMUS   H. Dietl and A. Philippu

In anaesthetized cats a push-pull cannula (Philippu et al., Naunyn-Schmiedeberg's Arch. Pharmacol. 276:103, 1973) was stereotaxically inserted into the posterior hypothalamus which was superfused with artificial cerebrospinal fluid (CSF) pH 7.2 at a rate of 0.15 ml/min. The superfusates were collected every 15 min for 6 h into tubes kept on dry-ice. The CSF contained pargyline (10^{-4}M), the tubes 50 μl EDTA (final concentration 10^{-3}M).Noradrenaline (NA), adrenaline (A) and dopamine (DA) were determined in the superfusates by a modification of the method of Da Prada and Zürcher (Life Sci. 19:1161,1976), GABA by the method of Enna and Snyder (J. Neurochem. 26:221,1976).
The spontaneous release was in the first sample (pmoles/15min; n=10-14, mean values $\pm$ S.E.M.): A 2.5$\pm$0.4, NA 3.1$\pm$0.5, DA 66$\pm$15, GABA 1312$\pm$229. The spontaneous release of A remained constant during the experiment, while that of NA, DA and GABA declined (24th sample: A 2.3$\pm$0.8, NA 2.4$\pm$0.7, DA 24$\pm$6, GABA 883$\pm$156).
Pretreatment of the cats with reserpine (1 mg/kg) virtually abolished the spontaneous release of catecholamines and strongly diminished that of GABA. Superfusion of the hypothalamus with KCl (100 mM) caused a pronounced enhancement of the release of all neurotransmitters. Electrical stimulation of the locus coeruleus increased the release of A, NA and GABA while the release of DA was not influenced.

Department of Pharmacology and Toxicology, University of Würzburg, Versbæcher Landstr. 9, D-8700 Würzburg

234

STUDIES ON THE EFFECTIVENESS OF DOPAMINERGIC SUBSTANCES ON THE EXPERIMENTALLY INDUCED MUSCULAR RIGIDITY OF RATS K. Halbhübner, and D. Loos

Reserpine as well as 6-aminonicotinamide (6-AN) are able to induce in rats an experimental rigidity which is demonstrable electromyographically and is used as test model for possible antiparkinson drugs (B.E. Roos, G. Steg, Life Sci. 3, 351, 1964; I. Jurna, G. Lanzer: Naunyn-Schmiedebergs Arch. Pharmak. exp. Path. 262, 309, 1969; H. Herken et al., Naunyn-Schmiedeberg's Arch. Pharmacol. 293, 249, 1976). We could demonstrate resp. confirm the dose-dependent effectiveness of the dopaminergic substances bromocryptine (H. Corrodi et al.: J. Pharm. Pharmac. 25, 409, 1973; A.M. Johnson et al.: Experientia 29, 763, 1973) and lisuride (R. Horowski, H. Wachtel: Europ. J. Pharmacol. 36, 373, 1976; W. Kehr: Europ. J. Pharmacol. 41, 261, 1977) on the electromyographically measurable muscular rigidity (J.M. Vigouret et al.: Naunyn-Schmiedeberg's Arch. Pharmacol. 297, R 54, 1977). The doses to reduce the spontaneous activity for the reserpine model ranged from 1-25 μg lisuride/kg and 59-750 μg bromocryptine/kg. For the 6-AN model 5-50 μg lisuride/kg and 500-10000 μg bromocryptine/kg i.p. are necessary. We obtained comparable results with 100 mg L-DOPA/kg in combination with the DOPA-decarboxylase blockers benserazide (peripheric effect, A. Pletscher, G. Bartholini: Clin. Pharmacol. Ther. 12, 344, 1971) and NSD 1015 (peripheric and central inhibition, A. Carlsson et al.: Naunyn-Schmiedeberg's Arch. Pharmacol. 275, 153, 1972) indicating the possibility of dopaminergic properties of L-DOPA itself.

Institut für Pharmakologie der Freien Universität Berlin, Thielallee 69/73, D-1000 Berlin 33

235

ATYPICAL NEUROLEPTICS: EFFECT ON DOPAMINE SYNTHESIS AND RELEASE IN RAT BRAIN IN VIVO   W. Kehr

Classical neuroleptics of the phenothiazine or butyro phenone type are known to block dopamine (DA) receptors and to stimulate DA synthesis and release via a negative receptor-mediated feedback mechanism. It was of interest to study the effect of chemically different compounds like clozapine, sulpiride, metoclopramide and rolipram (a new pyrrolidone derivative) on DA synthesis and release.
The accumulation of dopa after decarboxylase inhibition with 3-hydroxybenzylhydrazine was used as a measure of DA synthesis and the formation of 3-methoxytyramine (3-MT) after MAO inhibition with pargyline was taken as an indicator of DA release.
There was a marked and dose-dependent increase in striatal and mesolimbic dopa as well as 3-MT formation by haloperidol, pimozide and metoclopramide. With regard to 3-MT formation a maximum was reached at 0.2, 1 and 3 mg/kg i.p. of haloperidol, pimozide and metoclopramide, respectively. At higher doses of pimozide and metoclopramide 3-MT formation was reduced to half maximum values. Clozapine, sulpiride and rolipram stimulated dopa and 3-MT formation only at high doses whereas low doses (0.5-3 mg/kg i.p.) reduced the formation of 3-MT indicating decreased release of DA into the synaptic cleft.
The reduced activity of the dopamine neurons induced by the latter compound may contribute to or even be the cause of their neuroleptic profile.

Dept. Neuropsychopharmacology, Schering AG, Müllerstr. 170-178, D-1000 Berlin 65

236

INHIBITION OF LOCOMOTOR ACTIVITY OF RATS BY LOW DOSES OF DIFFERENT DOPAMINE (DA) RECEPTOR AGONISTS H. Wachtel

Apomorphine-HCl (APO) or the ergot derivative lisuride hydrogen maleate (LHM), both supposed to stimulate directly DA receptors, were injected subcutaneously to male Wistar rats (80-100 g). Immediately following the drug or vehicle application locomotor activity of individual rats was recorded during 10 min time intervals for 30-240 min using circular photocell motility meters. APO or LHM had a biphasic action on locomotor activity; in low doses (0.006-0.1 mg/kg) they caused hypomotility, while doses > 0.1 mg/kg produced motor stimulation. The suppression of motor activity induced by 0.1 mg/kg of APO or by 0.025 mg/kg of LHM was followed by hyperactivity; LHM caused a more pronounced and more long-lasting stimulation.
The stimulatory effect of 0.39 mg/kg of APO or LHM also occurred after the combined pretreatment with reserpine (7.5 mg/kg i.p., 4 h) and α-methyl-p-tyrosine (250 mg/kg i.p., 3.5 h). While the hyperactivity induced by APO or LHM could be antagonized by pimozide (6.25 mg/kg, 30 min), the hypomotility could partially be reversed by sulpiride (6.25 mg/kg i.p., 30 min).
The data further support the view of a direct dopaminergic action of LHM. The suppression of motor activity induced by low doses of APO or LHM is discussed in regard of hypothesized DA autoreceptors mediating inhibition.

Dept. Neuropsychopharmacology, Schering AG, Müllerstr. 170-178, D-1000 Berlin 65

237

THE EFFECT OF EMD 25 004 (5-methyl-3-/2-(4-phenyl-1,2,3,6-tetrahydropyridyl-1)-ethyl/-pyrazole) ON CENTRAL MONOAMINERGIC NEURONS
C.A. Seyfried and K. Fuxe

EMD 25 004, a novel psychotropic drug (5-methyl-3-/2-(4-phenyl-1,2,3,6-tetrahydropyridyl-1)-ethyl/-pyrazole), induces contralateral turning behavior in rats with unilateral, 6-hydroxy-dopamine induced lesions in the S. nigra without eliciting stereotyped behavior. In whole rat brain, EMD 25 004 (2.5 and 5 mg/kg i.m.) decreases the rate of dopamine (DA) depletion following catecholamine synthesis blockade by H44/68 (α-methyl-tyrosine), indicating a reduced central DA-turnover, whereas the rate of noradrenaline (NA) depletion is increased at a threshold dose of 0.5 mg/kg i.m., suggesting an increased NA-turnover. Furthermore, EMD 25 004 antagonises the serotonin (5HT) release induced by H75/12 (4-methyl-α-ethyl-m-tyramine) and decreases 5HT-utilisation in doses down to 2 mg/kg, as evidenced by a decreased rate of 5HT-depletion following 5HT-synthesis blockade by H22/54 (α-propyl-dopacetamide). It is concluded that EMD 25 004 directly stimulates central DA-receptors at least partially whereas 5HT-receptors are indirectly activated by inhibition of neuronal 5HT-reuptake. In contrast, NA-receptor activity is possibly reduced due to postsynaptic blockade. Because of possible more selective dopaminergic actions on the nigro-striatal system, EMD 25 004 may be useful in the treatment of extrapyramidal disorders.

Med. Research Dept., E. Merck, Darmstadt, and Dept. of Histology, Karolinska Inst.,Stockholm

238

THE EFFECTS OF BENZOCTAMINE (TACITIN[R]) ON REFLEXLY ACTIVATED γ-MOTONEURONES OF DECEREBRATED OR SPINALIZED CATS. E.F. Coelle, Hildegard Cremer, N.N. Osborne, K.-H. Sontag.

The concentration of dopamine and noradrenaline are decreased to a maximum of 40 % and 20 % respectively in the substantia nigra of precollicular and prenigral decerebrated cats previously treated with benzoctamine (0.7 mg/kg i.v.), while the tyrosine-hydroxylase and MAO activities remain unchanged. Muscle stretch reflexes recorded similtaneously showed a significant decrease of stretch tension which is avoked by a clear reduction of Ia dischanges of the primary muscle spindle afferents in decerebrated cats. In contrast the muscle tension in spinalized cats is slightly deminished and not accompanied by a reduced γ-activity. These results will be discussed in relation to γ-motoneurones being controlled by the supraspinal descending catecholaminergic nigro-spinal pathway. A decrease in the catecholamine content inhibits static γ-motoneurones whereas dynamic ones are excited.

Max-Planck-Institut für experimentelle Medizin, Hermann-Rein-Straße 3, D-3400 Göttingen (G.F.R.)

239

FORMATION OF ß-CARBOLINES: A NEW METABOLIC PATHWAY OF INDOLES IN THE BRAIN OF RATS
H. Rommelspacher, and B. Greiner

Several authors were able to show formation of ß-carbolines in vitro when indolealkylamines were incubated with 5-MTHF and homogenates from various tissues e.g. brain, blood platelets and heart. The products of the reaction inhibit high affinity uptake of serotonin and noradrenaline and to a lesser degree that of dopamine, choline and GABA. In pharmacological experiments the ß-carboline tetrahydronorharmane (THN) exerts serotonin-like activity and inhibits the action of apomorphin, a stimulant of dopamine receptors.
We now present data demonstrating substantial concentrations of THN in rat brain, blood platelets, and urine. The identity of the substance was shown by TLC in several solvent systems, two different co-cristallisation methods, and mass-spectrometry. Furthermore we have good evidence that 6-OHTHN, the derivative of serotonin occurs in vivo as well. The amount excreted by the urine is increased after treatment with phenobarbital. Since the compound crosses the blood-brain-barrier it can be expected that it is present in the CNS, too. 6-OHTHN is inactivated by conjugation with glucuronide. Whether 6-OHTHN is formed from serotonin directly or by hydroxylation of THN remains to be elucidated. In conclusion the present data demonstrate for the first time the existence of a derivative of tryptamine and serotonin with biological activity in vivo. Thus,a second pathway for indolealkylamines can be assumed besides oxidation by monoamineoxidase.

Institute of Neuropsychopharmacology, Free University of Berlin, Ulmenallee 30, D-1000 Berlin, West Germany

240

EXTRACTION OF COMPOUNDS WITH OPIOID ACTIVITY FROM MILK   H. Teschemacher, V. Brantl, and I. Haarmann

Recently, opiate-like behaving compounds have been detected in the blood, which seem to differ considerably from endogenous opioids identified so far. In view of the possibility that such opioids might pass from blood into milk either by passive diffusion or even by secretion, we searched for these opioids in human and bovine milk.
Chloroform/methanol extracts of lyophilized milk showed opioid activity in opiate receptor binding assays and in the guinea pig ileum longitudinal muscle/myenteric plexus preparation. These extracts contained several compounds with opioid activity as seen when the extracts were subjected to various chromatographic procedures. Like those opioids found in the blood, the opioids extracted from milk proved to be resistant to pronase, which might indicate that they are no peptides - in contrast to all endorphins identified so far. Maximum amounts of these opioids were found in winter, whereas in summer, during periods up to several months, they could not be demonstrated in the milk.
Such opioids might be ingested with milk or milk products; however, when recovered from that organism, by which, thus, they have not been produced, they have to be regarded as exogenous opioids; in such a case, "exorphins" might be their appropriate description.

Department of Neuropharmacology, Max-Planck-Institute for Psychiatry, Kraepelinstrasse 2, D 8000 München 40

241

RADIOIMMUNOASSAY (RIA) OF ß-ENDORPHIN
V. Höllt, Ch. Gramsch, and R. Przewłocki

The existence of several endogenous peptides
with opiate-like activity requires a specific
and sensitive method for their determination.
Therefore, we developed a RIA for ß-endorphin.
The antisera were obtained from rabbits which
had been injected with thyroglobulin-coupled
ß-human(h)-endorphin as immunogen. ß-h-endorphin
was isolated with ^{125}Iodine using chloramine T
as an oxidizing agent. The titer of the selected
antiserum was about 1:100 000. The sensitivity
of the RIA for ß-h-endorphin was in the range of
10 to 20 fmole per assay tube. The antiserum re-
cognized ß-camel-endorphin with the same avidity
as ß-h-endorphin. ß-h-lipotropin had a 2 fold,
γ-endorphin a 500 fold and α-endorphin a 3000
fold lower affinity than ß-h-endorphin. Methio-
nine-enkephalin had no affinity. This indicates
that the antiserum recognizes the C-terminal regions of ß-endorphin. Using this assay, we were
able to measure ß-endorphin-immunoreactivity in
separate areas of brain and pituitary glands, as
well as in the blood and cerebrospinal fluid of
man. In the blood of rats we found elevated ß-
endorphin levels both after adrenalectomy and
treatment with metyrapone. A similar finding was
obtained after different stress conditions (electrical footshock, insulin shock). Enhanced ß-endorphin levels were also seen in humans with
Cushing-Syndrome. We studied the release of ß-endorphin from rat pituitaries in vitro and found
an enhanced release by potassium and various hypothalamic extracts.

Department of Neuropharmacology, Max-Planck-
Institute for Psychiatry, Kraepelinstrasse 2,
D 8000 München 40

242

**PEPTIDASE-RESISTANT ENDOGENOUS LIGANDS FOR THE
OPIATE RECEPTORS**   R. Schulz, M. Wüster,
H. Schneider, and P. Loth

The identified endogenous ligands for the opiate
receptors (endorphins) are penta- and oligopep-
tides. Information recently accumulated from
several laboratories, including our own, suggest
the existence of endogenous opiate-like acting
material distinct from the peptide endorphins.
One of the main differences of this material
from the peptides appears to be its resistance
to various proteolytic enzymes, including pronase P. In addition, the material reported here
is of highly lipophilic character and behaves
like a cation, as indicated by its migration on
paper-electrophoresis at pH 2.0. Its biologic
activity is neither affected by exposure to cy-
anogen bromide nor to nitrous acid. However,
several properties of our material differ from
those of other endogenous, non-peptide opioid
compounds reported by other laboratories. The
peptidase resistant material described by Gintz-
ler et al. (PNAS 73, 2132, 1976) binds to morphine antibodies, migrates like morphine on thin-
layer-chromatography (TLC), but does not exert
opiate-like acting properties on the electrically stimulated guinea pig ileum. In contrast, our
material does not bind to morphine antibodies,
behaves differently from morphine on TLC, and
displays naloxone-reversible activity on the
isolated guinea pig ileum and mouse vas deferens.
Just how much these differences can be attributed to purification remains to be elucidated.

Supported by Deutsche Forschungsgemeinschaft.

Department of Neuropharmacology, Max-Planck-
Institute for Psychiatry, Kraepelinstrasse 2,
D 8000 München 40

243

**THE RELEASE OF ENKEPHALINS FROM RAT STRIATAL
SLICES IN VITRO**   H. Osborne

Several lines of investigation point to the possibility that enkephalins may function as neuro-
modulator/neurotransmitter agents in the mamma-
lian central nervous system. In this study we
report on the release of met- and leu-enkephalin
immunoreactivity from rat striatal slices in
vitro and on the effects of ions and opiate anal-
gesics on their release. 500-600 mg wet weight
striatal slices were superfused with oxygenated
Krebs-bicarbonate medium. Following lyophiliza-
tion, the samples were submitted to analysis by
a radioimmunoassay which exhibits a high degree
of specificity for met- and leu-enkephalin as
described previously (Wesche et al., Naunyn-
Schmiedeberg's Arch. Pharmacol., in press). The
spontaneous release of met- and leu-enkephalin
increased 7-10 fold in response to 50 mM potassium. The potassium-evoked release of enkephalin
was abolished in a calcium-deficient (0.1 mM)
and magnesium-rich (7.0 mM) Krebs medium. At the
end of the experiments, between 80-85% of the
initial met- and leu-enkephalin contents were
recovered in the slices; 25-30% of the decrease
in tissue enkephalin content could be accounted
for in the samples. Preliminary studies with
morphine (10^{-5}M) and naloxone (10^{-6}M) indicate
that these compounds have no effect on the release of enkephalins.

Department of Neuropharmacology, Max-Planck-
Institute for Psychiatry, Kraepelinstrasse 2,
D 8000 München 40

244

**EVIDENCE FOR A ROLE OF ENDORPHINS IN EMOTIONAL
HYPERTHERMIA**   J. Bläsig, and A. Herz

Little is known about the physiological role of
endorphins. In view of the effects of opiates on
body temperature a role in thermoregulation has
to be considered. This has prompted experiments
in which the effects of various endorphins on
core temperature were studied in rats and compared with the effects of opiates after intracerebroventricular or systemic administration (in
case of the endorphins only the enkephalin derivative FK 33 824 could be tested upon systemic
administration). Both groups of drugs induced
hyperthermia after low dosages and hypothermia
after high dosages, the former being present at
dosages considerably lower than those necessary
to induce analgesia (vocalization test after
electrical tail stimulation). Hyperthermia may,
therefore, be a primary action of the opioids, of
significance for the physiological role of endorphins.
Core temperature in rats is rather labile and can
be easily effected by manipulation, even slight
handling inducing an increase of more than 1°C.
This increase could be partially prevented by
systemic application of the specific opiate antagonist naloxone. After development of hyperthermia naloxone induced a dose-dependent decrease in core temperature, whether administered
systemically or intracerebroventricularly.
The non-availability of the (+)stereoisomer of
naloxone did not allow testing of the specificity of this naloxone effect. The above findings,
however, strongly suggest a participation of
endorphins in emotional hyperthermia.

Department of Neuropharmacology, Max-Planck-
Institute for Psychiatry, Kraepelinstrasse 2,
D 8000 München 40

245

ANTAGONISM BY OPIATES AGAINST PROSTAGLANDIN E$_2$-STIMULATED ADENYLATE CYCLASE IN THE CORPUS STRIATUM   K. Kuschinsky and U. Havemann

The actions of opiates on the elevation of cyclic AMP (cAMP), induced by prostaglandin E$_2$ (PGE$_2$), were studied in slices of the rat striatum. Morphine (2μM) antagonized the PGE$_2$-induced elevation of cAMP, while an equimolar concentration of naloxone inhibited morphine's effect. The action of morphine was mimicked by met-enkephalin (100μM, in presence of 0.2 mM bacitracin) and by levorphanol (10μM), but not by an equimolar concentration of its stereoisomer dextrorphan. Adenosine (1mM) or an elevation of K$^+$-ions to 54 mM raised the cAMP concentration, and PGE$_2$ induced a further elevation, which however, was not antagonized by morphine under these conditions.
6 days after injection of kainic acid (1μg) into the striatum, the stimulation by PGE$_2$ of adenylate cyclase was even enhanced, while the stimulation by dopamine of this enzyme was lowered. These results suggest that the PGE$_2$-stimulated adenylate cyclase is mainly localized in nerve endings of afferent neurones. The cell bodies of them are located outside the striatum. In striata, lesioned by kainic acid, morphine did not significantly antagonize the PGE$_2$-induced stimulation. Therefore, the involved opiate receptors are probably located on neurones, the cell bodies of which being within the striatum and not on endings of afferent neurones.

Abt. Biochemische Pharmakologie, Max-Planck-Institut für Experimentelle Medizin, Hermann-Rein-Str. 3, D-3400 Göttingen

246

QUANTITATIVE EVALUATION OF THE MORPHINE ABSTINENCE SYNDROME IN MICE AND THE INFLUENCE OF SOME ANTAGONISTS OF THE CNS TRANSMITTERS ON THE WITHDRAWAL SIGNS.
B.-D. Görlitz

Morphine pellets prepared according to Gibson and Tingstad(J.Pharm.Sci.,59,426,1971) containing different doses of morphine base (10-100 mg) were implanted s.c. in mice to produce dependence on morphine. The abstinence syndrome was produced by i.p. injection of 4 mg/kg naloxone. The following signs were evaluated: "jumping"(dominant sign),"wet dog shaking"(recessive sign),defecation and urination.The observation of these symptomes in mice allowed a better quantification of dependence,similar to the results of Bläsig et al. in rats(Psychopharmacology,33,19,1973).A dose of 50 mg morphine resulted in a high degree of dependence and a distinct abstinence syndrome produced by naloxone.Higher doses showed no advantage; stress and lethality however are enhanced.- The used antagonists of the CNS transmitters(given 30 min. before naloxone) showed different influences on the abstinence signs. Phenoxybenzamine(5 mg/kg p.o.) and haloperidol (1mg/kg i.p.) caused a decrease of all abstinence signs. The 5-HT antagonist cyproheptadine (0.5 mg/kg i.p.) enhanced the abstinence syndrome; atropine(1.5mg/kg p.o.) blocked only the recessive wet dog shaking. As a central depressant drug pentobarbital (30 mg/kg i.p.) was used,which could block the wet dog shaking. It is apparent that the physiological basis of dependence on morphine and the abstinence syndrome is localized mainly in brain regions where the catecholamines and 5-HT act as transmitters.

Med.-Vet. Klinik I, Justus-Liebig-Universität Giessen D-6300 Lahn-Giessen, Frankfurter Str. 126

247

PROVOKED AND SPONTANEOUS WITHDRAWAL IN THE DETERMINATION OF DEPENDENCE ON MORPHINE
M. Fernandes, and S. Kluwe

To clear the relationship between provoked and spontaneous withdrawal the intensity of both was determined in the rat after identical schedules of morphine (M.) administration (2 x 16 mg/kg or 2 x 32 mg/kg M.-HCl daily). In experiment I dose-response realtionships (DRR) of naloxone-HCl were determined before and 4 hours after the morning injection (32 mg/kg) on day 1, 5, 10, and 20 of treatment. The following symptomes were observed: jumping, writhing, wet dog shake, diarrhea, body weight loss, ptosis, and scream on touch. With exception of an increase of writhing on day 20, the DRR´s were identical on day 5, 10, and 20. In comparison to pre-M. -withdrawal four hours after M. jumping was intensified, ptosis not altered, and all other symptomes decreased. In experiment II it was shown that the DRR´s of naloxone were strongly dependent on the last dose of M. When elevated to 32 mg/kg (in 2 x 16 mg/kg M. -treated rats on day 10) they could not be distinguished from those obtained in 2 x 32 mg/kg treated animals. In experiment III spontaneous withdrawal was observed in 2 x 32 mg/kg M. -treated rats after 5, 10, and 20 and in 2 x 16 mg/kg M- treated animals after 10 treatment days. The rats did not show significant hyperalgesia (hot plate and tail flick) nor hyperthermia. The results of food and water intake were complicated by direct effects of M. The body weight loss was identical in 2 x 32 mg/kg treated rats but significant less after the lower chronic dose of M. The results show that spontaneous and provoked withdrawal do not develop completely in a parallel manner.

Institute of Neuropsychopharmacology, Free University of Berlin, Ulmenallee 30, D-1000 Berlin, West Germany

248

INFLUENCE OF DRUGS ON ESCAPE BEHAVIOR FOLLOWING DIFFERENT KINDS OF AVERSIVE STIMULI IN RATS OF DIFFERENT AGE.
N. Steiner, and G. Schulze

Rats are able to modify ambient temperature (a.t.) by an operant behavior which is thermoregulatorily relevant.
As shown elsewhere (SCHULZE,G., P.BÜRGEL, Naunyn Schmiedeberg´s Arch.Pharmacol, 298, 143-147(1977)) the behavior elicits different a. t. depending on the following variables: a) preset a.t., b) age of the animal, and c) application of the drug which influences body temperature, e.g. phentolamine.
In order to test whether these variables influence the behavioral reaction via specific thermoregulatory functions or via unspecific aversive stimulus escape the following experiments were carried out. Groups of rats of different age (6-8 months and 26-30 months) were trained on a classical shock (foot shock) escape schedule. Trained animals were then subjected to a schedule of stepwise increased shock intensities (16 steps). Lever pressing terminated the shock and reset the shock to minimal intensity. The average shock intensity to which the rats responded was determined and compared. Old rats show a more sensitive response both in cold as well as in shock escape behavior. In both age groups phentolamine increases escape reaction against cold stimulus and decreases the reaction against foot shock. Morphine decreases the escape reaction against both kinds of aversive stimuli. Therefore one may assume that the two drugs influence operant behavior on different levels of specificity.

Institute of Neuropsychopharmacology, Free University of Berlin, Ulmenallee 30, D-1000 Berlin, West Germany

249

TETRAHYDRONORHARMANE (THN) AND 6-HYDROXY-NORHARMANE: PHYSIOLOGICAL COMPONENTS IN PLATELETS AND URINE OF MAN. H. Honecker, and H. Coper

Tryptamine as well as 5-hydroxytryptamine are metabolized by monoamineoxidase. On the other side the compounds can also react with formaldehyde to form the condensation products THN and 6-OH-THN. There is little information about the presence of these substances in the organism and about their physiological significance, particularly because no sensitive analytic method existed to determine the quickly oxydable compounds. With a new radiometrical procedure (Honecker and Rommelspacher, 1978) measuring even 1 ng THN and 6-OH-THN the existence of the derivatives in the urine and platelets of man was investigated. It could be proved that THN is eliminated with the urine. The night sample contained approx. 40 ng with a great interindividual deviation. After treatment with 4 g tryptophan the evening before collecting, the amount of urine-THN increases 40 fold. 6-OH-THN can be detected in the urine, too. So far, no quantitative determination has been performed. Similar results were found in platelets. Compared to serotonin, the THN-content of the platelets is small (1ng/10^8 platelets) but increased 10 fold after loading with tryptophan. In serum normally no THN or 6-OH-THN can be detected, after load with tryptophan a certain amount has been found occasionally. Therefore it seems likely, that THN and 6-OH-THN are stored in platelets in a similar way as serotonin.

Institute of Neuropsychopharmacology, Free University of Berlin, D-1000 Berlin , Ulmenallee 30, West Germany

250

INCREASE IN SENSITIVITY OF THE FLUOROMETRIC PLASMA HISTAMINE DETERMINATION: ROUTINE ASSAY IN THE FEMTOMOL RANGE W. Lorenz, B. Schöning, B. Schwarz, and E. Neugebauer

Our fluorometric histamine assay was sensitive enough to differentiate 100 pg/ml plasma from blanks, but the VC % was more than 10% in the subnanogram range. Thus histamine release in sepsis, polytrauma, ileus etc. could not be determined with a sufficient precision. For this reason the sensitivity of the method (W. Lorenz et al., Z.Physiol.Chem. $\underline{355}$, 1097, 1974) was enhanced by changing the reaction conditions and by lowering considerably the blanks.
Condensation run for 40 min. at 0° C. 0.2 ml M HCl was added (final pH 2.2 - 2.3, n=10). Millipore$^{(R)}$ water was used. 5 M and 0.1 M NaOH (both salt-saturated) were treated by n-butanol, n-heptan (Uvasol$^{(R)}$, Merck) was purified by 0.1 M HCl. oPhthaldialdehyde (Fluka) was recrystallized slowly at 21° C. The Zeiss spectrum fluorometer (ZFM$_4$C) was equipped with a HTV R 446 photomultiplier, the slit widths were kept as small as possible.
Using this procedure 20 pg histamine/ml plasma could still be differentiated from blanks. For pool plasma obtained from 140 orthopedic patients (280 pg histamine/ml) the VC % was only 6.9% (n=15). In 10 of these subjects single values of 70, 105, 160, 160, 225, 230, 240, 500, 650 and 930 pg/ml were determined which were in agreement with previously published plasma histamine values.

Department of Experimental Surgery, University of D-3550 Marburg (Lahn), Robert-Koch-Straße 8

251

RENAL EXCRETION OF D-GLUCURONIC ACID METABOLITES AS A MEASURE FOR MICROSOMAL ENZYME INDUCTION B. Roth, E. Gladtke

Under clinical conditions the direct biochemical measurement of xenobiotic enzyme induction in liver microsomes is not possible. But the renal excretion of metabolites of the hepatic D-glucuronic acid pathway can be used as a measure for drug related induction of microsomal liver enzymes. The renal excretion of D-glucaric acid is enhanced in humans during treatment with many drugs (J.Hunter et al., Lancet $\underline{I}$,572,1971). Studies in rats show that renal excretion of xylitol indicates hepatic microsomal enzyme induction too (B.G.Lake et al., Toxicol.Appl.Pharmacol. $\underline{35}$,113,1976).
In 70 children of different age the quantitative excretion of D-glucaric acid and xylitol was determined in urine of a 24-hour collection period. D-glucaric acid shows a characteristic diurnal rhythm with maximal excretion in the early afternoon and minimal in the night. Newborn show no characteristic diurnal variations in D-glucaric acid excretion. The diurnal rhythm develops in the first weeks of life.
After therapeutic treatment of jaundiced newborn with 7.5mg/kg phenobarbitone for 5 days renal D-glucaric acid excretion was increased from o.12 ±o.o5 μM/d to 1.08±o.34 μM/d (n=11). Xylitol excretion was also found increased.
Children during anticonvulsive therapy show an average D-glucaric acid excretion of 5.5 μM/d in contrast to o.9 μM/d in untreated children. The excretion of xylitol increased in a similar pattern. Enhanced renal excretion of both metabolites could observed from 48 to 72 hours after initial treatment until 8 days after therapy.

Children's Hospital, University of Cologne, GFR D5 Köln 41, Josef-Stelzmann-Strasse 9

252

PHARMACOKINETICS OF FENTANYL - EVALUATION OF AN INFUSION MODEL J.H. Hengstmann, H. Stoeckel, and J. Schüttler

An intravenous infusion scheme can be established on the basis of pharmacokinetic analysis that allows a smooth clinical analgesia for the entire duration of surgery.
Concentrations of fentanyl were measured by RIA (Michiels et al. Europ.J.clin.Pharmacol. 12,153, 1977). After a bolus injection serum levels were declining with a half-life of 1 to 2 minutes followed by a slower ß-phase (t/2 2 hours). The volume of the central compartment was equal to the plasma volume. The transfer constant (k 12 = 0.59) considerably exceeded the elimination rate constant (kel = 0.13).
In most patients, however, an increase of serum levels could be seen between 1 and 2 hours after injection. Shortly after injection fentanyl was measured in gastric juice with high levels. A complete enteric absorption was demonstrated following oral ingestion of fentanyl. This supported the hypothesis that fentanyl is secreted into the stomach and reabsorbed from the gut.
Neglecting the amount reabsorbed the infusion model was developed as described by J.G. Wagner (Clin.Pharmacol.Ther. 16,691,1974) on the basis of an open two-compartment model.
The comparison of EEG background activity and serum levels made it necessary to maintain during the infusion equilibrium a serum level of 15 to 20 ng/ml for "medium" pain level and 20 to 25 ng/ml for laparotomy.
This aim could be achieved by this infusion model.

Department of Internal Medicine, University of Bonn, D 53 Bonn 1, Venusberg

253

A METHOD FOR MEASURING PLASMA PROTEIN BINDING OF TRICYCLIC PSYCHOACTIVE DRUGS AT THERAPEUTIC LEVELS

M. Brinkschulte, I. Jahns, and U. Breyer-Pfaff

By reacting the corresponding primary or secondary amine analogues with ^{3}H-methyl iodide, the following drugs were synthetized at specific radioactivities of 1-7 Ci/mmol: amitriptyline (AT), nortriptyline (NT), imipramine, desmethylimipramine, perazine, and clozapine. The drugs were isolated by thin-layer chromatography and their purity was frequently checked with this technique. They were added to human plasma or albumin solutions at varying concentrations, the lowest being 10 ng/ml (appoximately $3 \cdot 10^{-8}$M). Equilibrium dialysis was carried out in Teflon^R cells separated by Visking cellulose membranes (Bickel and Steele, Chem.-biol. Interactions $\underline{8}$, 151, 1974) against phosphate-buffered saline. Under these conditions, adsorption of drugs to the apparatus amounted to only 10-15 % even with low quantities added. Equilibrium was achieved within 6 hr at 37°C, and tritium concentrations were measured in both half-cells.

Using low concentrations of AT and NT, the free fractions were found to comprise around 4 and 9 %, respectively, in plasma from AT-treated patients as well as from healthy volunteers. Likewise, the free perazine fraction (2-3 %) did not differ between a group of patients receiving the drug and healthy controls. There were, however, single values which considerably deviated from the average, particularly with AT.

Scatchard plot analysis of AT and NT binding disclosed the occurrence of at least two sets of binding sites, one of these exhibiting high affinity and low capacity. Binding to this site became apparent only with drug concentrations below $5 \cdot 10^{-5}$ M. The same applied to solutions of human serum albumin, and here the capacity of the high-affinity site was found to be 0.1-0.2 mol/mol. Albumin, however, differed from plasma in binding NT more firmly than AT.

Department of Toxicology, University of Tübingen, Wilhelmstr. 56, D-7400 Tübingen

254

INVESTIGATIONS ON DPH PROTEIN BINDING

A.Haass, K.W.Pflughaupt, and A.Schütz

Generally in clinical practice only the total plasma concentration of anti-epileptic drugs and not the unbound fraction is measured. For highly protein bound drugs as DPH(Diphenylhydantoin) this would be sufficient if the proportion of the unbound fraction is nearly the same in all patients. But large and small variations in the extent of DPH plasma protein binding have been reported.

The aim of the present study was to determine the variation of the bound:unbound ratio dependent upon the DPH plasma level and the plasma albumin concentration. DPH was bound in a constand proportion over a large range of the total plasma concentration (nearly $10^{-6}-10^{-4}$ M) which included the therapeutic range. The binding constant was estimated as $1,5 \times 10^4$ $1 \times Mol^{-1}$. There seemed to be two protein binding sites in the therapeutic range.

We found a good correlation between plasma albumin concentration and the ratio of protein bound DPH. $8,6 \pm 0,4$ % of the DPH was bound with small individual variations in cases of normal albumin concentration. But this ratio increased up to 3 times of the normal value with decreasing albumin concentrations. The investigation of PORTER et al.(1975) of a small number of patients showed a linear relationship between the albumin concentration and DPH binding, whereas our results lead to a hyperbolic function. From the curve obtained the free fraction which correlates with the antiepileptic effect and the development of toxicity, could be determined in a sufficiently precise way in most of the patients, who had known albumin concentrations.

Depart.of Neurology, 87 Würzburg, J.Schneider-Str.

255

THE INFLUENCE OF PLASMA LEVEL MONITORING OF ANTIEPILEPTIC DRUGS ON THERAPEUTIC OUTCOME IN EPILEPTIC OUTPATIENTS. PART 1: STUDY DESIGN

R. Gugler and H. Penin

Although plasma level monitoring of antiepileptic drugs is commonly accepted as means to achieve better seizure control, no controlled clinical trial has yet been reported to demonstrate the benefit of routine plasma level monitoring. A study was designed in which 127 epileptic outpatients were randomly allocated to Group A (treating neurologist received results of plasma levels; dosage was adjusted by combined use of this information with all results of history, clinical and EEG findings), or to Group B (dosage was adjusted by use of history, clinical and EEG findings only). Only patients were included who had a minimum of 3 seizures over the preceding year. Patients were seen regularly at 3 months intervals over a total period of one year. The number of seizures as well as the frequency of drug related side effects was used to evaluate the effect of plasma level monitoring. The patients were informed on the fact that plasma levels were determined. In Group A it was attempted to have the plasma level within the therapeutic range if clinical data did not suggest different doses. The drugs determined were carbamazepine (& epoxide metabolite), phenobarbital, phenytoin, primidone, ethosuximide, sodium valproate. The therapeutic concentrations were as defined by Kutt and Penry (Arch. Neurol. $\underline{31}$, 283, 1974). 105 patients completed the trial: 21 with grand mal seizures, 53 with grand mal seizures and psychomotor seizures, 31 with grand mal seizures and absences.

Departments of Medicine and Neurology, University of Bonn, 53 Bonn - Venusberg

256

THE INFLUENCE OF PLASMA LEVEL MONITORING OF ANTIEPILEPTIC DRUGS ON THERAPEUTIC OUTCOME IN EPILEPTIC OUTPATIENTS. PART 2 : RESULTS

M. Eichelbaum and W. Fröscher

No significant differences could be observed in therapeutic outcome between patients of group A and B. In both groups of patients the number of seizures decreased during the study year as compared to seizure frequency of the preceeding control year. The decrease of seizure frequency was accompanied by an increase of plasma concentrations of antiepileptic drugs. The number of patients with all antiepileptic drugs monitored in the therapeutic range increased in both groups from 45 % to 56 %. There was no difference in drug treatment between the two groups. The number and kind of drugs administered were similar in group A and B. Drug treatment did not change substantially during the study as number and kind of drugs administered to treat the patients was very similar at the beginning and end of the study. Drug compliance was not different in group A and B. In both groups the incidence of side effects were similar. During the study the number of side effects decreased . Common side effects as fatique, headache, and dizziness did not correlate with drug plasma levels. Only for phenobarbital such a correlation was observed . There was, however, a positive correlation between plasma levels and the development of ataxia.

A positive correlation could be observed between increasing plasma levels and slowing of EEG background activity.

In conclusion, under the conditions of the study knowledge of plasma levels of antiepileptic drugs did not further improve antiepileptic therapy.

Departments of Medicine and Neurology, University of Bonn, D 5300 Bonn - Venusberg

257

PHARMACIKINETICS OF CARBAMAZEPINE AND ITS ACTIVE METABO-
LITE, CARBAMAZEPINE-1o,11-EPOXYD AFTER SINGLE AND CHRONIC
ADMINISTRATION IN HEALTHY HUMANS.   M. Sigmund, G.Heimann,
and M. Theisohn

The antiepileptic carbamazepine (CARB) is a strong inducer
of its own metabolism. As the main metabolite, carbamaze-
pine-1o,11-epoxyd (EPOX) has similar antiepileptic potency,
the kinetics of CARB and EPOX were studied in healthy volunteers receiving CARB per os as a single dose (11mg/kg)
and thereafter chronically during 15 days (8mg/kg.day).
During the acute trial blood was collected three times a
day. During the chronic medication blood was drawn every
second day and after the last dose for 1 week 3 times a
day. Urine was collected in day portions during the whole
time. Serum and urine levels of CARB and EPOX were determined by HPLC using a RP-8 column, methanol-water eluent
and absorption measurement at 215 nm. Pharmacokinetic calculations were carried out with a digital computer assuming an open-one-compartment model for CARB and EPOX and
first order kinetics of the absorption of CARB and the metabolic production of EPOX. From the data of the acute
trial the following parameters were estimated for CARB:
distribution coefficient=o.74-o.98 1/kg (assuming complete
intestinal absorption), absorption rate=o.1-o.4 h^{-1}, elimination rate=o.o18-o.o32 h^{-1}; for EPOX: production rate
=o.o48-o.o78 h^{-1}, elimination rate=o.o2o-o.o32 h^{-1}. CARB
and EPOX were eliminated unchanged in small quantities
via the kidneys (1% each). After the chronic treatment
the elimination rate of CARB and EPOX were increased by
about 7o and 1oo% resp. Parallel to the increased elimination there was a small decrease of the serum levels of
CARB and EPOX and a pronounced reduction of the side
effects after 1o days of medication. As a sign of increased hepatic metabolism the glucaric acid content of
the urine was augmented 15-5o fold. Hence, CARB induces
the metabolism and elimination of its metabolites, too,
which might be responsible in part for the side effects.
Depart.of Pharmacol.,D5ooo Cologne 41, Glueeler Str.24

258

ANTICOAGULANT ACTIVITY OF THE ENANTIOMERS OF ACENO-
COUMAROL IN MAN   T. Meinertz, W. Kasper, E. Jähnchen,
J. Godbillon, and J. Richard

For the mono-coumarin derivatives warfarin and phenprocoumon it was shown that in man and rats the S(-)
enantiomer is several times more potent as anticoagulant
than the R(+)enantiomer. These stereoselective differences in the anticoagulant potency reflect differences
in the affinity for the receptor site rather than differences in the pharmacokinetics.

In 4 healthy volunteers we have studied the anticoagulant
activity and the plasma concentrations of the enantiomers
of acenocoumarol following single i.v. injections of
0.25 mg/kg. Acenocoumarol differs from warfarin only by
a nitro-group in para position of the phenyl ring. Opposite to the results reported for warfarin and phenprocoumon, R(+)acenocoumarol was several times more potent
as anticoagulant than S(-)acenocoumarol. Plasma concentrations of R(+)acenocoumarol were considerable higher
than those of S(-)acenocoumarol. From these findings it
appears that the stereoselective differences in the anticoagulant activity of acenocoumarol in man could result
primarily from stereoselective differences in the disposition of acenocoumarol.

II. Medizinische Klinik und Pharmakologisches Institut
der Universität Mainz; Ciba-Geigy Biopharmaceutical
Research Center, Rueil-Malmaison, France.

259

HPLC-DETERMINATION OF SULFAPYRIDINE AND ITS METABOLITES IN
HUMAN PLASMA AND ITS PHARMACOKINETICS IN MAN C.Fischer
and U.Klotz

For the treatment of Crohn's disease and ulcerative colitis
salicylazosulfapyridine(SASP)is a drug of first choice.One
of the active moities is sulfapyridine(SP).Acetylation
rate to its major metabolite N-acetylsulfapyridine(AcSP)is
genetically controlled and a therapeutic range of 20-50µg
totalSP/ml was postulated.We developed a HPLC-assay to measure in plasma simultaneously SP,AcSP and the 5-hydroxyla-
ted metabolite(SPOH) to determine the phenotype and the
plasma levels of patients treated with SASP.Additionally,
the disposition of SP was investigated in 4 healthy volunteers after a single oral dose of 4g SASP and 1.25g SP.
100-200µl plasma, 500µl acetate buffer(pH4.7) and the internal standard sulfadimidine were extracted with chloro-
form.The organic phase was evaporated to complete dryness
and the residue was redissolved in methanol/water(20/80).
The different compounds were separated within 10-15minutes
on a 10µm Nucleosil RP-18 column by eluation with methanol/
1% acetic acid(20/80).From the 38 patients tested 19 subjects could be regarded as slow acetylators.In 13 patients
plasma levels were in the toxic range.After the single
oral dose of SASP SP could be detected in plasma after a
lag time of 6h.Thereafter maximal plasma levels between10
and 30µg/ml were reached within 27hrs.Elimination became
predominant after about 24h with a T1/2 of 12.6+6.4(mean+
SP).Following the direct administration of SP the drug
could be detected in plasma after 0.5h and absorption rate
was fast(k_a=1.0h^{-1}).Elimination of SP could be characterized by a T1/2 of 10.9+4.8h and a total plasma clearance
of 82+75ml/min.In no case free SPOH could be detected.The
concentrations of AcSP varied dependent on the phenotype
between 5 and 15µg/ml.Since side effects are almost exclusively directed to slow acetylators if plasma levels are
above 50µg/ml,measurements of SP and AcSP by our fast and
specific assay may help in improving therapy with SASP.
Dr.Margarete Fischer-Bosch Institut für Klinische Pharmakologie Auerbachstr.112, D-7000 Stuttgart 50

260

PREOPERATIVE HAEMODILUTION AND THE ACTION OF
NEUROMUSCULAR BLOCKING AGENTS   F.T. Schuh

The clinical concept of normovolemic haemodilution (HD) and
autologous blood re-transfusion is now accepted as a safe and
effective method to reduce the administration of homologous bank
blood and the incidence of serum hepatitis. To study the influence
of HD on the action of muscle relaxants during neuroleptanaesthe-
sia, in a group of 47 surgical patients two units of venous blood
were withdrawn preoperatively and replaced by 1000 ml of dextran 40. Haemoglobin and haematocrit changed from 14.2 ± 1.6
to 10.7 ± 1.5 g/100 ml resp. from 41.4 ± 3,8 to 31.4 ± 3.7%,
total serum protein from 7.1 ± 0.4 to 5.3 ± 0.6 g/100 ml, and
serum cholinesterase (ChE) from 5.8 ± 0.9 to 3.6 ± 0.9 U/ml.
Neuromuscular blockade was quantitized by means of mechano-
grams of the hand muscles after supramaximal electrical stimulation of the ulnar nerve. 34 patients without HD served as controls. – Following HD the potency of d-tubocurarine (dTC),
pancuronium (PC), and suxamethonium (SuM) was increased as
shown by cumulative dose-response curves which displayed a
parallel shift to the left, the ratio ED_{50} control/ED_{50} HD being
2.1 (dTC), 2.5 (PC) and 2.7 (SuM). Accordingly, the
duration of action of a single ED_{90} of dTC (0.21 mg/kg), PC
(0.033 mg/kg), and SuM (0.3 mg/kg) was prolonged 1.4 – 1.8
times after HD.–
The increased potency and duration of action of neuromuscular
blocking drugs following HD is thought to be due 1) to a rise of
cardiac output and skeletal muscle perfusion, 2) to a decrease of
binding to serum protein, and 3) in the case of suxamethonium to
a lowered hydrolytic activity of serum ChE.

Supported by Deutsche Forschungsgemeinschaft.
Dept. of Anaesthesiology, University of Kiel, D 23 Kiel
Hospitalstrasse 40

261

CARBONIC ANHYDRASE INHIBITORS AS BRONCHOLYTIC SUBSTANCES. W.K.R. Barnikol and K. Diether

Broncholytic substances decrease the bronchial tone and therefore the anatomical dead space volume (VD). This was shown in case of atropine by Severinghaus and Stupfel (J.Appl.Physiol.8,81,1955). The method of Fowler was used. We have developed a new method for measuring the anatomical dead space, which is also applicable in case of lung desease (Barnikol, Diether : Pneumonologie 152, 227, 1975 ; Barnikol, Diether, in preparation). The anatomical dead space volume can be measured breath by breath. With the new method first the bronchial actions and reactions in time and second by variation of tidal volume (VT) the VD-VT-relation can be measured. The slope of this relation is a measure for the bronchial compliance. Application of fenoterol to lung healthy people results in an increase of both, anatomical dead space (30 ml) and bronchial compliance. With the aid of our new method we have reinvestigated the influence of CO_2 on the bronchial system. In literature there are discrepancies (Stein et al.,Resp.Physiol.25,363,1975; Widdicombe, Physiol.Rev.43,1,1963 ; Barer et al., Bull.Physiol.Path. 8,459,1972). Some authors find bronchodilation, others bronchoconstriction after application of CO_2.

Our measurements show, that after an inspiratory jump of CO_2 concentration from 0 to 3.4 Vol% initially a bronchodilation occurs. At the same time big oscillations are seen (so called bronchial peristalsis). By the time (10 min) on the average the bronchodilation is compensated and bronchoconstriction occurs. So both groups of the authors mentioned above were right. From these experiments we conclude, that CO_2 naturally is a stimulus for the bronchial tone. Therefore carbonic anhydrase inhibitors were believed to have a broncholytic effect. By experiments this was verified : after inhalative application of diamox, methazolamide and dichlorphenamide in healthy people the anatomical dead space increases to the same extent as in case of fenoterol.

Physiologisches Institut, Universität, Saarstr. 21, 65 Mainz, BRD

262

HEMODYNAMIC EFFECTS OF ACUTE β-ADRENERGIC BLOCKAGE WITH ATENOLOL Gerloff,J. Bodem,G, Ochs,H.R. Czypionka,M.

8 healthy volunteers (age 25±4 years) received in randomized sequence 50, 100, 200, 400, and 600 mg Atenolol orally and 50 mg Atenolol intravenously during 5 minutes under continuous ECG monitoring. On 3 consecutive days prior to the first application of Atenolol the volunteers were exercised on the treadmill under continuous measurement of the blood-pressure until a heart rate of 150 min[1] was achieved. This individually determined load was used on the treadmill 3 h after oral and 1 hour after i.v.-application of Atenolol.Systolic and diastolic blood pressure and heart rate was measured at rest and after 1.5 min and 3 min of exercise. The results are expressed as difference between rest (=0) and exercise in blood pressure (Δs=systolic, Δd=diastolic RR in mm Hg) and heart rate (HR in min[-1]).

		control	Atenolol in mg oral 50	100	200	400	600	i.v. 50
1.5	Δs	0	-7,63	-17,96	-27,40	-25,24	-32,40	-24,18
min	Δd	o	6,43	-2,60	-6,32	-11,89	-16,40	-8,08
	HR	0	-26,76	-28,66	-29,41	-33,16	-34,66	-32,76
3	Δs	0	-9,27	-24,93	-31,73	-27,34	-36,01	-29,76
min	Δd	0	-4,35	-1,23	-7,81	-12,81	-16,00	-10,38
	HR	0	-29,83	-31,33	-32,57	-35,08	-39,33	-35,58

To determine the degree of β-adrenergic blockage before and 3 hours after Atenolol Isoproterenol was applied as bolus injection in consecutively higher dosage to mark off the dosage of Isoproterenol necessary to increase the heart rate by 30 min[-1]. The required amount of Isoproterenol(in ug) is shown below

Atenolol(mg)		i.v.	oral				
	control	50	50	100	200	400	600
Isoproterenol	3,5	10,13	9,38	18,5	31,75	55,25	94

Medizinische Universitätsklinik , University of Bonn
D 5300 Bonn 1 - Venusberg

263

HALOTHANE-INDUCED LIPID PEROXIDATION IN MAN AND RAT AS MEASURED BY ETHANE FORMATION IN VIVO, V. Hempel, U. Köster

Lipid peroxidation in vivo can be demonstrated by the measurement of ethane formation (Riely et al., Science 183, 208, 1974; Köster et al., Toxicol. Appl. Pharmacol. 41, 639, 1977). Ethane is measured by gas chromatography.

Rats exposed to halothane breathing a concentration of 2 % in pure oxygen were found to produce about 6 nmol ethane per kg body weight and hour, compared to about 12 nmol/kg/h when dosed with 1 g/kg carbon tetrachloride. These results stimulated us to measure the ethane content in the expiratory air of patients before and after clinical anaesthesias with halothane. In nine of 24 patients after halothane anaesthesia a significant increase of the ethane concentration in the range of 40 - 170 % could be demonstrated, compared to none in a control group of 12 patients which underwent a neuroleptanalgesia. None of the "halothane-responders" showed evidence of liver damage in the postanaesthetic period. The formation of ethane during halothane anaesthesia is considered to be due to reactive intermediates which occur during halothane biotransformation. The halothane-induced lipid peroxidation may give rise to sensitization reactions against chemically altered lipid structures of liver cells, thus causing liver damage.

Zentralinstitut für Anaesthesiologie und Institut für Toxikologie der Universität Tübingen, D 7400 Tübingen

264

ELIMINATION OF PARATHION BY HEMOPERFUSION IN SEVERE E 605 FORTE[R] INTOXICATION IN VIVO S. Okonek

Severe parathion (P) intoxication results in complete inhibition of cholinesterase activity and toxic accumulation of acetylcholine. Besides these well known biochemical changes, there is evidence of d i r e c t toxic effects on the cardio-vascular system which may prove fatal due to an excess of P.

Causal therapy aims at eliminating P, and hence reducing its concentration in blood and tissues. Hemoperfusion (H) with coated activated charcoal has proved to be sufficient in eliminating P from the blood in vitro.

In in vivo trials two groups (2 x 4) of mongrel dogs rereived 3o mg P per kg body weight i.v.. Both groups were treated symptomatically. One group was additionally treated by a 4 hour-hemoperfusion.The resulting P clearance values were 81.ol $\pm$ 18.17 ml/min. P blood levels in both groups similary decreased from about 4ooo ng/ml to 552 $\pm$ 195 ng/ml and 657 $\pm$ 16o ng/ml (controls) respectively 8 hours after injection. The concentrations of P in the muscles however were reduced 3 hours after beginning of H to 4.2 $\pm$ o.5 µg per g wet weight and 6.1 $\pm$ o.9 µg per g w.w. (controls) respectively; the corresponding values after 4 hour-hemoperfusion were 3.5 $\pm$ o.6 and 5.9 $\pm$ 1.1 µg per g w.w.. 8 hours after the injection the animals were sacrificed. The P conc. in the brain was found to be 3.8 $\pm$ o.7 and 5.2 $\pm$ o.7 µg per g w.w. (controls) respectively.

In the blood of two patients who suffered from severe E 6o5 forte[R] intoxication after an attempt to commit suicide hemoperfusion clearance values were determined, which were similar to those described in the animal experiments. Tissue conc. of P in man are not yet avaiable intra vitam, but the reduced P tissue concentrations in the animals favours H in severe P intoxication in man.

Centre Detoxication and Poisons Information,
II. Med. Clin. University of Mainz, Langenbeckstrasse 1
W-Germany

265

Carbromal - a "sedative" of similar potency to barbiturates   H.-W. Vohland, Th. Schirop

In humans acutely poisoned with carbromal(=CAL) the serum contains CAL (2oo-3oo µmoles/l) and its two metabolites bromoethylbutyramide (=carbromide=CID, 3oo-4oo µmoles/l) and ethylbutyrylurea(=EBU, 4o- 6o µmoles /l).The clinical signs of central nervous system depression correlate well with the serum concentrations of CAL and its two metabolites.
In rats the pharmacological activity of CAL, CID and EBU was examined and compared with that of phenobarbitone (=PB). Following i.p.injection, the LD-5o values were found to be 1,8 mmoles/kg CAL,1,5 mmoles/kg CID, 5 mmoles/kg EBU and o,9 mmoles/kg PB.After injection of an anesthetic dose righting refex returned at brain concentrations of 33o nmoles/g CAL, 56o nmoles/ g CID, 89o nmoles/g EBU and 336 nmoles/g PB. The protective activity against pentetrazol induced generalized convulsions was nearly identical for CAL, CID and PB but 2-3 times less with EBU.CAL, CID and PB severely decreased body temperature. Hypothermic activity of EBU was found to be weak. On isolated fundus strips CAL,CID and PB were able to reduce tone and strength of contraction elicited by acetylcholine, 5-hydroxytryptamine, histamine or $BaCl_2$ at nearly equal molar concentrations.
The findings show that CAL is metabolized in humans to considerable amounts of the pharmacologically active metabolites CID and EBU. The activity of CALand of CID was found to be qualitatively and quantitatively similar to that of PB.
Institut für Toxikologie und Pharmakologie der Universität Marburg, Pilgrimstein 2, D- 355o Marburg

266

DEPENDENCE ON 2,2 DIETHYL-4-PENTENAMIDE (DIETHYL-ALLYLACETAMIDE, IN NOVO-DOLESTAN[R], INSOMNIA[R])
W.Poser, C.Speer, B.Kellermann, and S.Poser

19 patients with a chronic abuse of 2,2 diethyl-4-pentenamide(DEP) have been observed in a two years period(1976/77). The majority had been dependent on alcohol or bromoureides before their abuse of DEP, but cases of primary DEP abuse also occured. The patients reported an increase in dose of DEP up to 4,5 g/day. It occured within a few days in dependents on other substances of the alcohol-barbiturate group. During intoxication we observed inactivity, hostility, ataxia, dysarthria and nystagmus in patients. Withdrawal symptoms consisted of anxiety, tremor, sweating, grand mal seizures and delirium tremens. They could be relieved by clomethiazol(Distraneurin[R]) or diazepam(Valium[R]). The majority of patients felt addicted to DEP. During intake of DEP an elevation of gamma-glutamyltransferase in serum occured, but GOT(aspartate aminotransferase), GPT(alanine aminotransferase), alkaline phosphatase and bilirubin remained normal. This pattern may be helpful in the follow-up of patients at risk.

We conclude that DEP causes drug dependence similar to that on alcohol or barbiturates. It is used as an alternative to other substances like alcohol or bromoureides. It may lead to a rapid relapse in persons prone to drug dependence. As DEP is available without prescription in the BRD a rapid increase of chronic abuse may be expected as soon as bromoureides have become prescription drugs.

Psychiatrische und Neurologische Universitäts-kliniken, 34 Göttingen, v.Sieboldstr. 5

267

PRESENT DRUG SITUATION   G.Müller

The illicit drug market is determined by heroin. There are also large amounts of cannabis.-Over all the drug criminality increases since 1972. Wanke (Pharmazeut.Z.122,1o54,1977) names 4o.ooo addicts as the hard core. The number of drug deaths increases every year. The German heroin market has changed during 1977. Southeast Asia heroin (Nr.3):3o-4o% heroin,3o-4o%caffeine,1% acetylcodein, 1% strychnine and barbital a.o. has been replaced by Near and Middle East heroin ("turkish heroin"):7o-8o%heroin,2-6%acetylcodein and traces of narcotine and papaverine.Some samples contain the alkaloids partly as free bases.We distinguish between different types.-Addicts often think heroin contains very toxic compounds.Strychnine f.i.is added during manufactoring in small amounts.The reason may be a better flavour during smoking.Heroin Nr.3 is originally a smoking material.The assumption strychnine is nessecary for the bitter taste of bad mixtures is not correct.-Recently severe convulsions during heroin injektions has been reported.(Loos,Crime Dept.Frankfurt)The reason may be mixtures with phenazon.-Cocaine is not very important at this moment.-Beside cannabis only amphetamines have some importance.Recently a very dangerous hallucinogene 4-bromo-2,5-dimethoxy-amphetamine has appeared.(Hall,CID-Lab. Frankfurt)-There are some other drugs with small and more local importance.-Cannabis and opium surrogates have been seen.The wide spread misuse of tilidin (Valoron[R]) is reported.

Hessisches Landeskriminalamt, Dept.IV/2
Hoelderlinstr.5, D-62oo Wiesbaden